Anaesthesia and the E.M.O. System

Other books of interest

Anaesthesia, Recovery and Intensive Care
D. A. Buxton Hopkin, M.D. (Lond.), F.F.A.R.C.S.
Consultant Anaesthetist, Charing Cross and St. Thomas' Hospitals, London.

Principles of Intensive Care
E. R. J. Emery, M.B., Ch.B., F.F.A., R.C.S., D.A.
Consultant Anaesthetist, Charing Cross Hospital, London.
A. K. Yates, M.B., Ch.B., F.R.C.S.
Consultant Thoracic Surgeon, Guy's Hospital, London.
P. J. Moorhead, M.B., Ch.B., M.R.C.P.
Consultant Physician, Northern General Hospital, Sheffield.

A Short Textbook of Medicine
J. C. Houston, M.D., F.R.C.P.
Physican and Dean of the Medical and Dental Schools, Guy's Hospital, London.
C. L. Joiner, M.D., F.R.C.P.
Physician, Guy's Hospital, London.
J. R. Trounce, M.D. F.R.C.P.
Professor of Clinical Pharmacology and Sub-Dean of the Medical and Dental Schools, Guy's Hospital, London.

A Short Textbook of Preventive Medicine for the Tropics
A. O. Lucas, M.D., D.P.H., D.T.M.&H., F.R.C.P., S.M.Hyg., F.M.C.P.H.
Professor of Preventive and Social Medicine, University of Ibadan .
H. M. Gilles, M.D., F.R.C.P., M.F.C.M., M.F.C.P.H., D.T.M.&H.
Professor of Tropical Medicine, Liverpool School of Tropical Medicine.

Urgencies and Emergencies for Nurses
A. J. Harding Rains, M.S., F.R.C.S.
Professor of Surgery, Charing Cross Hospital Medical School.
Valerie Hunt, S.R.N., S.C.M., R.N.T.
Principal, The United Sheffield Hospitals School of Nursing.
Margaret D. Mackenzie, S.R.N., S.C.M.
formerly Ward Sister, Charing Cross Hospital, Fulham.

Films about the E.M.O. system
The E.M.O. and constant low concentration anaesthesia (1962).
Clinical use of the E.M.O. inhaler (1963).
Technique of ether anaesthesia (1964).
Intercostal block (1963).

These are available through Penlon Ltd., formerly the Longworth Scientific Instrument Co., Radley Road, Abingdon, Berks., England.

Anaesthesia and the E.M.O. System

JOHN V. FARMAN, F.F.A.R.C.S.,
Consultant Anaesthetist, Addenbrooke's Hospital, Cambridge

HODDER AND STOUGHTON
LONDON SYDNEY AUCKLAND TORONTO

ISBN 0 340 16700 9

First printed 1973
Reprinted 1980

Text set in 10/11 pt. IBM Press Roman, printed and bound in Great Britain
at The Pitman Press, Bath
for Hodder and Stoughton Educational,
a division of Hodder and Stoughton Ltd.

Acknowledgments

Acknowledgments and thanks are due to all those who assisted in the preparation of this book. To Mrs. Marian Allen for her excellent illustrations; to Sir Robert Macintosh, the late Dr. Denys Waters, Dr. Edward P. Dosher, Dr. I. Wakai and Mr. Neville Ripley for reading and criticising the manuscript; to Mr. Anthony Jephcott, Mr. B. R. Sugg and Mr. Neville Ripley of the Longworth Scientific Instrument Co. for their technical advice, criticism and encouragement; to the Editors of *Anaesthesia, British Medical Bulletin, Acta Anaesthesiologica Scandinavica,* and the *Journal of the American Medical Association* for permission to reproduce illustrations which first appeared in their journals; to Mr. Leonard Beard and members of the Department of Medical Illustration, Addenbrooke's Hospital; to the Longworth Scientific Instrument Company and British Oxygen Company for the use of some of their illustrations; to Miss Jean Dickens, Mrs. Ann White and Mrs. Grace Ashton for typing the manuscript; to all those doctors, nurses, and technicians who tolerated my eccentricities in the operating theatres at University College Hospital, Ibadan, Baptist Medical Centre, Ogbomosho, Wesley Guild Hospital, Ilesha, Cardiff Royal Infirmary, Zaria General Hospital and Addenbrooke's Hospital, with such patience and helpfulness.

This book is dedicated to all doctors and their assistants working in small hospitals, often in remote and difficult conditions, for whom anaesthesia represents a dangerous and worrying procedure.

Contents

Chapter One

Introduction

The need for anaesthesia is world-wide and by no means confined to the
large and expensively equipped hospitals of rich industrial societies. In
tropical countries the pattern is usually that of a few big hospitals and a
larger number of much smaller hospitals, each with only one or two doctors
(Farman, 1962b, 1968). Money for equipment may be short or facilities
limited and the doctor may be assisted in the operating theatre by a nurse
or may be entirely on his own. Such conditions are found in thousands
of small rural hospitals throughout the world. The same considerations also
apply to the giving of anaesthetics in domiciliary practice, on expeditions,
on board ship, in civil disasters and major accidents, in time of war or
whenever electricity, medical gas supplies and water are cut off and skilled
personnel are not available (O'Connor, 1961; Temmerman, 1960;
Macintosh and Parkhouse, 1961; McNally et al., 1962; Boulton, 1966).

These situations have in common the absence of trained anaesthetists
(who naturally congregate in the large hospitals), shortage of money
(because even rich countries are reluctant to put aside equipment for
emergency use) and often the need for portability. It follows from this
that any method employed should be simple, portable, cheap and above
all safe. In many instances these criteria can be adequately met by the
use of local or regional anaesthesia. However, there are many operations,
such as those about the head and neck, chest operations and upper
abdominal operations, for which local anaesthesia is inappropriate. There
are also many patients, particularly children and very ill patients, who
tolerate regional techniques badly. General anaesthesia, on the other hand,
is of almost universal applicability. The advantages are that the patient
is spared much avoidable distress and time is saved in comparison with
extensive local techniques. However, certain requirements must be met
if general anaesthesia is to be given safely. The concentrations and doses
of drugs given must be known, it must be possible to give artificial
respiration if breathing fails and to pass an endotracheal tube. At the same
time, the apparatus must be simple enough to be easily understood by
the non-specialist and cheap enough to be universally available (Macintosh,
1955; Farman, 1971).

The techniques described in this book are based on the work of Sir

Robert Macintosh and his colleagues at Oxford (Parkhouse and Simpson, 1959). They have developed a system of anaesthesia employing air as the carrier gas, with temperature compensated vaporisers for volatile anaesthetic agents. The system is based on the use of ether, which is unique among general anaesthetics in that it can actually stimulate both respiration and the circulation, making it possible to employ air, whereas most general anaesthetics need to be used in conjunction with oxygen. For this reason it has proved the safest anaesthetic agent, even in the hands of inexpert anaesthetists. Snow (1848) believed it almost impossible for death to occur from ether administered with ordinary intelligence and attention.

The E.M.O. inhaler (designed by Dr. H. G. Epstein, physicist in the Oxford Department and Professor Macintosh at Oxford) is recognised as the best so far designed.

It is the most widely used of a long line of draw-over anaesthetic vaporisers, the first of which was described in 1846. A simple glass inhaler with a non-return valve was used by Morton to give the first successful ether anaesthetic at Boston in that year. Similar devices were used in London a few weeks afterwards. In 1847 Snow designed an inhaler which enabled the concentration to be controlled, but in spite of this good start, little further development of vaporisers took place for many years. At the beginning of the twentieth century, interest revived when the need for an accurately calibrated chloroform vaporiser became apparent. This development was, however, soon overshadowed by the introduction of compressed gas anaesthetic machines. In spite of many advantages, some of these were complicated and badly designed, allowing rebreathing or presenting the patient with a high resistance. They all had in common the disadvantage that it was impossible to determine the concentration of vapour that the patient was receiving.

In 1937 Sir Robert Macintosh was appointed Professor of Anaesthetics at Oxford University. He was at that time concerned about the increasing dependence of anaesthetists on their complex apparatus which he determined to simplify. He emphasised the importance of delivering a known concentration of vapour while at the same time reducing the size and complexity of the machines themselves (Macintosh, 1955). In 1941 Epstein, Macintosh and Mendelssohn described the famous Oxford Vaporiser which achieved wide popularity all over the world. It was a portable ether inhaler with a temperature regulating device. The E.M.O. itself was introduced by Macintosh and Epstein in 1952 as a successor to the Oxford Vaporiser. Since then various accessories have been developed in order to extend its range of usefulness, notably the Oxford Miniature Vaporiser (O.M.V.) and the Bryce-Smith Induction Unit (B.S.I.U.). It is possible to combine the various vaporisers, bellows, valves and oxygen flowmeter unit in different ways, so as to make a number of 'anaesthetic machines', to suit the special

needs of individual doctors or hospitals (see Chapter 6). For this reason
the term 'E.M.O. System' is used in this book. It is truly modular and
has proved highly versatile. Recently a number of similar systems, employing draw-over vaporisers for inhalational agents, have been introduced. They
have been reviewed by Boulton (1966), but it is fair to say that the E.M.O.
system is by far the most successful.

The E.M.O. system has an additional role as a teaching aid. Because it
has only essential controls, it is conceptually simple, consisting of a series
of units each of which has a well defined purpose. It is useful for teaching
medical students, particularly in countries where graduates will be expected
to work on their own in small hospitals and who will have to supervise the
work of nurse or medical assistant anaesthetists. It also has a role in a more
sophisticated environment, as an insurance against a disaster situation. It
is the author's opinion that all specialist anaesthetists should be able to use
the system.

In many of the situations described above the doctor is working on his
own and naturally feels obliged to do the operation himself. If this is so,
it will clearly be necessary for him to delegate at least part of the anaesthetic
to an assistant (Rigg, 1961; Webb, 1968; Boulton, 1966) who may be
another doctor, a nurse or medical assistant or even a layman. The expertise
possessed by these people will vary enormously, from none at all to a
considerable level of competence, and the only safe course is for the doctor
in charge to be thoroughly conversant with the type of anaesthetic
employed. This means that he must himself learn how to give anaesthetics so
that he will be in a position to supervise his assistant and to instruct and
help where necessary. In most circumstances, it will be the doctor who
actually induces anaesthesia, probably passing an endotracheal tube,
before handing over to the assistant. He will then be free to scrub up and
perform the operation. At the end of the operation he will actively
supervise extubation and emergence from anaesthesia.

Although this book is written primarily for doctors, it is hoped that it will
also prove useful to medical students, nurses and medical assistants whose
job it is to assist with or even to give anaesthetics.

Anyone who gives anaesthetics should have some knowledge of anatomy
and physiology, in order to appreciate the importance of fluid balance,
respiration and the circulation of the blood, and of pharmacology in order
to understand the complex effects of anaesthetic drugs. For this reason
chapters on physiology and pharmacology relevant to anaesthesia have
been included in this book, although it is appreciated that for many
readers they will merely serve as reminders of well known facts. An assistant
should of course know how to maintain a clear airway in an unconscious
patient. He should be able to detect and count the peripheral pulse and to
take the blood pressure. He should understand the purpose and method
of functioning of the apparatus. He should be a methodical person capable

of making sure that all likely instruments are within reach before the start of the anaesthetic, and of keeping an accurate record of the anaesthetic. Many assistants will have been trained to do much more than this, but the doctor should never forget that the final responsibility for the anaesthetic is his (Rigg, 1961).

The specialist anaesthetist may be called upon in an emergency to give an anaesthetic outside the large hospital which is his normal habitat. Even these hospitals will occasionally be cut off from their normal supplies of gases and this will probably mean using unfamiliar draw-over apparatus for the first time. It is hoped that this book will be helpful to the specialist who is obliged, possibly at short notice, to learn these techniques. Lastly, a chapter on regional anaesthetic techniques has been included. The object has been to offer descriptions of all anaesthetic techniques likely to be required by the doctor working in a small hospital. Regional anaesthesia plays an important part in these circumstances, although on the whole unrelated to the E.M.O. system.

Clearly the principal object of anaesthesia is to enable operations to be performed without pain. It is sometimes forgotten that pain is not the only ill effect of surgery. The patient may suffer physiological derangements both during the operation and afterwards, and it is also the function of anaesthesia to protect him from these. At the same time the anaesthetic itself may have a marked effect on physiological function and it is important to limit this as much as possible. While the patient's comfort is essential, the most important consideration will be his safety, and there will be times when comfort appears to take second place to safety, particularly when life is in danger and time is short. Nevertheless, the greatest possible regard must always be paid to the feelings of the patient and even the simple methods advocated here will be acceptable if presented with gentleness and consideration.

Chapter Two

Physiology

In the normal subject the different physiological systems serve the needs of the organism as a whole. In man these needs are various and most systems have a considerable range of activity, the ultimate function of which is to keep constant the physical and chemical environment of the cells. In doing so, these systems interact so that, for example, in an anaemic patient the cardiac output increases, mitigating the effect of the reduced oxygen carrying capacity and maintaining the supply of oxygen to the tissues. In order to be able to do this, physiological systems rely on their reserve capacity and tend as a result of auto-regulatory, reflex or humoral mechanisms to adapt themselves to the increased functional loads placed upon them. In illness a patient is likely to suffer some disability which will interfere initially with at least one of these systems and will, if unchecked, end by interfering with all of them.

The most important systems from the anaesthetist's point of view are respiration and circulation. Firstly, these two systems are responsible for the transport of oxygen from the atmosphere to the tissues. Failure at any point along the way will deprive the tissues of their most essential fuel, resulting in anaerobic metabolism and finally cell death. Secondly, they are essential pathways for the uptake and distribution of anaesthetic drugs. At the same time, anaesthetic drugs themselves obstruct at least some sections of these pathways, so the anaesthetist must be aware at all times of the state of function of these systems in his patient, regulating the dose or concentration of drug used so as to produce only the desired effect. Neglect of these considerations, even by those whose knowledge and training should make them fully aware of them, has cost many patients' lives.

Fortunately, most of our patients are in reasonably good health and there is some margin of safety in the reserve capacity mentioned above. Di-ethyl ether, the agent advocated for general purposes in this book, actually stimulates both respiration and circulation in the majority of patients, at least under light surgical anaesthesia of the type recommended. In these patients, only mismanagement and lack of care can do harm, but when we meet severely ill patients, who lack physiological reserve, skill is required to steer the patient between too light a level of anaesthesia on the one hand, and respiratory or circulatory depression, leading to tissue hypoxia, on the other.

This chapter starts with a brief description of the important steps in the transport of oxygen to the tissues, mentioning how both anaesthesia and disease may affect them. A section on fluid and electrolyte balance follows.

Respiration

1) *The upper respiratory tract*

This is an often neglected part of the respiratory system. The nose warms, humidifies and filters the air. Whenever it is by-passed by an oral airway or endotracheal tube (i.e. during the majority of anaesthetics) the air entering the lungs will be at room temperature, unsaturated with water vapour (at body temperature) and possibly contaminated by dust or bacteria. These complications can be minimised by using a filter on the air intake to the vaporiser and by inserting a vapour condenser in the circuit when using an endotracheal tube.

The anatomy of the mouth, nose and pharynx is shown in section in Figure 2.1. The patient is in the supine position usually adopted during anaesthesia. Note that the soft tissues tend to fall backwards and to obstruct breathing. This is one of the fundamental complications of unconsciousness in general and anaesthesia in particular. Anaesthetics abolish protective reflexes and reduce muscle tone. The soft palate falls back, forming a valve which permits inspiration through the nose but prevents expiration. The mandible also drops back and the mouth falls open. The tongue is attached to the mandible via the hyoid bone and as a result, the tongue itself comes to rest on the posterior pharyngeal wall. This prevents air passing in either direction. However, tilting of the head (extending the atlanto-occipital joint) will raise the mandible and lift the tongue, usually restoring the airway. This is fully described in Chapter 5.

2) *The larynx*

This organ serves primarily as a sphincter to protect the trachea and lungs against aspiration of foreign matter. The anaesthetist's view of the larynx is shown in Figure 2.2. The upper part of the larynx consists of the epiglottis, aryepiglottic folds and the arytenoid processes. The two arytenoid cartilages are the key to the function of the larynx.

Attached to the arytenoids and passing forwards to the thyroid cartilage are the vestibular folds or false cords. These contract and come together during laryngeal spasm, effectively sealing off the larynx. This normally occurs during swallowing and prevents food and drink going down the wrong way. The space between the aryepiglottic folds and the false cords is the vestibule. The vocal cords lie beneath the false cords and are also

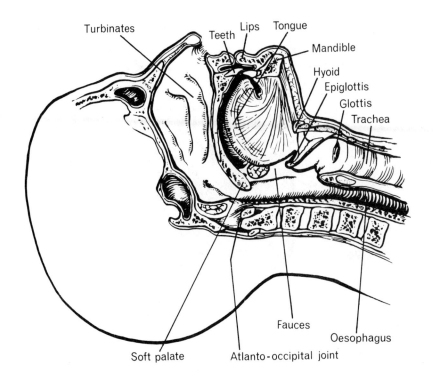

Fig. 2.1   Sagittal section of the head in the supine position to show the relationship of the mouth, nose and pharynx

attached to the arytenoid and thyroid cartilages. They move in phonation and contract during laryngeal spasm. The sphincter thus has two components. All anaesthetics in sufficiently large doses will stop it functioning but sometimes only at the expense of respiratory and circulatory depression. For this reason the anaesthetist commonly uses a muscle relaxant to paralyse the laryngeal muscles before passing an endotracheal tube (see Chapters 3, 5 and 7).

The glottis is the space between the vocal cords and is the narrowest point in the adult airway, but in children the cricoid ring is narrower. During intubation the tip of the tube may stick in the pyriform fossa (lateral to the aryepiglottic fold), the vestibule or in the saccule (above the true cords). Damage to the cords may be followed by the formation of a granulomatous polyp. Infections of the larynx and anaphylactic reactions are often accompanied by oedema of the arytenoids and false cords, which may

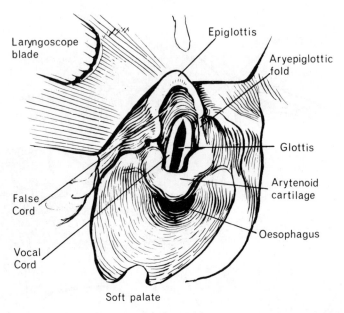

Fig. 2.2   Anaesthetist's view of the larynx (from a photograph taken with an Olympus fiberoptic endoscope)

completely obstruct the airway. The vocal cords themselves are seldom affected and it is usually possible to pass a small tube by gently advancing the tip between the oedematous false cords. Both the abductor muscles, which move the cords apart from each other, and the adductors which approximate them, are supplied by the recurrent laryngeal nerve. If this is injured abductor paralysis is more pronounced than adductor paralysis and as a result, the cords come to lie together, causing difficulty in speech and in breathing, evidenced by huskiness and stridor. During normal breathing the cords move apart on inspiration and come together on expiration. Spasm of the larynx is caused by irritant vapours, painful stimuli such as dilating the anal sphincter, and by the presence of foreign material.

3) *The trachea and bronchi*

The trachea is about 10 cm long in the adult and is supported anteriorly by cartilagenous arches which can often be seen in the relaxed patient with the aid of the laryngoscope. Ciliated mucosa is responsible for moving secretions upwards towards the glottis. The action of the cilia is said to be unaffected by ether, but depressed by cold and sedative drugs (Lee and

Atkinson, 1968). The cough reflex is active throughout the length of the trachea, but particularly at the carina (the division of the trachea into the two bronchi).

The right main bronchus in the adult is almost in line with the trachea, and a long endotracheal tube will therefore tend to pass into this side, preventing adequate ventilation of the left lung. Bronchi dilate on inspiration and constrict during expiration, constriction being caused by vagal activity, histamine, morphine and too light a level of anaesthesia.

4) *The lungs*

The function of the lungs is to transfer oxygen from the air via the alveoli to the blood, while at the same time carbon dioxide passes in the opposite direction. The respiratory system maintains normal levels of oxygen and carbon dioxide in the arterial blood. The former is essential for tissue metabolism, while control of the rate of excretion of carbon dioxide is an important short-term means of regulating the acid-base state of the body.

The volume of air taken into the lungs every minute (the Minute Volume) is around six litres in the resting adult, consisting of about twelve breaths of around 500 ml Tidal Volume (the volume of a single breath). About 150 ml of each breath fills the nose, trachea and bronchi (the Anatomical Deadspace), while the remainder enters the alveoli. The amount of air entering the alveoli every minute is known as the Alveolar Ventilation and is the product of the Tidal Volume (less the Deadspace Volume) and the frequency (number of breaths per minute) i.e. Alveolar ventilation = (Tidal volume − Deadspace volume) x frequency. A further small part of this air reaches alveoli which are not properly perfused with blood and so does not contribute to the exchange of gases. Normally less than one third of each breath is wasted in these ways (Deadspace Ventilation). This value remains the same in spontaneously breathing patients anaesthetised with ether and air (Marshall and Grange, 1966).

There are three ways in which oxygen uptake by the bloodstream becomes inadequate under anaesthesia even in normal patients. Firstly, the inspired air may contain too little oxygen. Secondly, the lungs may not be adequately ventilated, resulting in the perfusion of underventilated alveoli. Lastly, the circulation to the lungs may be impaired, resulting in ventilation of under-perfused alveoli. Although these three possibilities are considered separately as an aid to comprehension, it should be emphasised that pure defects of the types described seldom exist. Rather, combined deficiencies will be seen under clinical conditions.

a)   *Low inspired oxygen tension*
During anaesthesia with the equipment described in this book, the commonest cause will be the use of a high ether concentration. When

breathing 20 per cent ether, the maximum delivered by the E.M.O., the inspired oxygen concentration will be reduced to just over 16 per cent instead of the normal 21 per cent. At or near sea level the arterial tension will be reduced, but without significantly lowering the saturation, because of the shape of the oxy-haemoglobin dissociation curve. At high altitudes the inspired tension will already be low, and the use of 20 per cent ether will more rapidly lead to desaturation. This will represent a particular danger to patients whose oxygen transport is already impaired. The most vulnerable are those with sickle-cell disease, in whom the haemoglobin is rendered insoluble by exposure to low oxygen tensions. The treatment is to add oxygen to the inspired mixture (see Chapter 4).

b)   Underventilation of the lungs
This is frequently the result of respiratory obstruction, either due to disease or accompanying anaesthesia. Upper airway obstruction occurs as a result both of unconsciousness (see page six) and of organic obstruction of the upper respiratory passages. The signs are stridor (but only in the case of partial obstruction), tracheal tug with indrawing of the upper chest and later, cyanosis. Severe lower airways obstruction, accompanied by wheezing, may render a patient unfit for an inhalational induction with ether and air, although in many cases endotracheal intubation, followed by assisted respiration with ether and oxygen, will be beneficial. Many drugs will depress respiration, the most dangerous being the opioids which should only be used before anaesthesia for the treatment of pain. Central respiratory depression due to opioids is characterised by a reduced frequency of breathing with, at first a normal tidal volume, but later, the tidal volume is reduced and apnoea occurs. Barbiturates can also depress respiration and should therefore not be given before anaesthesia, but most of the newer tranquillisers are devoid of this undesirable side-effect. Curiously, the anaesthetised patient suffering from central respiratory depression is often able to cough even after breathing has ceased.

The effect of a period of suxamethonium-induced apnoea (total cessation of breathing) on arterial oxygen saturation was studied by Weitzner, King and Izekono (1959). They found that even after a period of moderate hyperventilation with air, the arterial oxygen saturation fell to around 60 per cent within 90 seconds. On the other hand, if the patient had been ventilated with 100 per cent oxygen for two minutes beforehand, the saturation did not fall significantly for over 120 seconds. Clearly periods of coughing or breath-holding during ether/air anaesthesia will be accompanied by low arterial oxygen tensions, unless oxygen has been added to the inspired mixture. Clearly also patients who are given muscle relaxants must be ventilated adequately (see Chapters 5 and 8).

Underventilation of the lungs may occur under anaesthesia even when relaxants are not used. In light anaesthesia most patients are capable of increasing the work of breathing to overcome the extra load imposed by increased airway resistance due to minor degrees of obstruction or reduced total compliance (Nunn and Ezi-Ashi, 1961; Scott and Slawson, 1968). Large abdominal tumours, ascites and external pressure on the chest or abdomen, such as found in the steep Trendelenberg or prone positions, will also increase the workload of breathing. However, deep levels of anaesthesia with ether will depress respiration (see Chapter 3) and should therefore be avoided even in the absence of these disabilities.

Other conditions which cause underventilation are pleural effusions, pneumothorax, hiatus hernia and massive collapse of the lung. Underventilation even of parts of the lungs will cause anoxaemia. In the case of collapsed or otherwise totally unventilated alveoli, although the blood flow will be reduced, a certain amount of perfusion will still take place. As a result, venous blood will pass through the lungs without taking part in gas exchange. This is known as venous admixture or right to left shunting.

Minor degrees of underventilation will respond initially to treatment with 100 per cent oxygen, but if prolonged will permit the arterial carbon dioxide tension to rise to a dangerous level. Major degrees will require artificial respiration (see Chapter 5). Further improvement will depend on removal of the causative factor.

c)   *Underperfusion of the lungs*
As almost the whole output of the heart passes through the pulmonary capillaries any factor lowering the output will reduce the pulmonary capillary flow.

Under normal conditions the mean pressure in the pulmonary arteries is about 20 cm H_2O. The actual pressures in the arteries will vary according to their positions, being lower in those above the level of the heart and vice versa. If the total flow is reduced (i.e. the cardiac output falls), the pressure will tend to fall and flow through parts of the lung may even cease altogether. However, these areas will continue to be ventilated, contributing to the physiological deadspace.

Treatment of underperfusion depends initially on the use of 100 per cent oxygen to raise the tension of oxygen in those alveoli that are adequately perfused. Artifical respiration will help if the patient is underventilating, but often he is already hyperventilating. Definitive treatment will depend on correcting the cause of the reduced cardiac output (see below).

Circulation of the blood

The main purpose of the circulation is to carry oxygen from the lungs to the tissues. It also acts as a transport system for carbon dioxide, products of digestion and hormones, and as a chemical and thermal buffering agent (Burton, 1965). However, this chapter will consider it only from the point

of view of the oxygen flux which is the total amount of oxygen carried
to the tissues in any period of time (Nunn and Freeman, 1964). Mathe-
matically it is the product of the cardiac output and the oxygen content
of the blood.

O_2 flux (ml O_2/minute) = Cardiac output (1/minute) x O_2 content

(ml O_2/minute)

The integrity of the oxygen flux will depend on an adequate volume of
blood, an adequate cardiac output, an adequate oxygen carrying capacity
and normal uptake of oxygen in the lungs. Although these aspects are
discussed separately it must be remembered that they interact with each
other, and that a change in any one of them will alter the others.

The blood volume

The body normally responds to a reduction in blood volume by increased
sympatho-adrenal activity, resulting in peripheral vaso-constriction and
redistribution of the cardiac output, which helps to maintain adequate
perfusion of the brain and heart. These reactions are accompanied by a
reduction in the urine output which conserves body fluid and by an increase
in alveolar ventilation which helps to maintain a normal arterial oxygen
tension. Meanwhile transfer of fluid from the tissue spaces into the bloodstream occurs, and the veins constrict, reducing the capacity of the
circulation. However, if a further reduction in blood volume occurs,
changes take place which indicate that the body has exceeded its ability
to compensate. The venous return to the heart is so reduced that the
cardiac output is no longer maintained and perfusion, even of vital organs,
becomes inadequate. At the same time the tissues extract more oxygen
from the blood so that the blood entering the lungs is desaturated and
severe arterial hypoxaemia may then follow impaired pulmonary gas
exchange. As a result the oxygen tension in the tissue cells falls to an even
lower level and anaerobic metabolism occurs. This leads to the production
of acid metabolites (metabolic acidosis) which, by their toxic effect on
the heart, further reduce cardiac output. Such a shocked patient will have
a rapid and possibly irregular pulse with a low blood pressure; his skin
will be pale and clammy; his mucosae will be a blue-grey colour and his
respiration will be depressed, with marked tracheal tug. Unless treatment
is given immediately, his heart will stop and he will die.

Factors affecting the blood volume

a)   Dehydration
This results either from a reduction in fluid intake or from excessive fluid
and electroloyte loss associated with vomiting, diarrhoea, or extensive
trauma, burns or peritonitis. The depletion of the blood volume in these

conditions will reflect a reduction in the extracellular fluid volume. Signs of dehydration are a dry mouth, thirst, oliguria, sunken eyeballs, shrunken tongue, reduced skin elasticity and eventually low blood pressure. If these signs are present a deficit of at least 5 per cent in extracellular fluid volume has occurred (Moyer, 1954). This is fully discussed at the end of this chapter.

b)   *Haemorrhage*

Blood loss during operation can be estimated by weighing the swabs on a 100 g spring balance and subtracting the weight of the same number of dry swabs. 1 gram of blood is equivalent to 1 ml. The loss of 10 per cent of the blood volume will cause moderate shock, while the loss of 40–50 per cent may be fatal.

c)   *Increased capacity of the vascular bed*

This is due to vasodilation and occurs in bacteraemic shock, heat-stroke and anaesthesia. The skin will be warm but if the circulation is sluggish, cyanosis will be present.

d)   *Pregnancy*

A 50 per cent increase in blood volume occurs in pregnancy.

e)   *Over-rapid infusion*

Over-rapid infusion of electrolyte solutions or blood will increase the blood volume and the venous pressure will rise.

Redistribution of the blood volume within the vascular space

This occurs under certain circumstances, for example vaso-vagal fainting. It may also follow the use of certain drugs which cause vaso-dilatation and postural hypotension. In this group are anaesthetics, some antihypertensives, some phenothiazines, and large doses of most sedatives and analgesics. Redistribution of blood is also caused by obstruction of the inferior vena cava, usually by an abdominal tumour. Blood tends to pool in the legs and pelvis, cardiac output drops and the heart rate rises. Blood pressure may fall. In late pregnancy, for example, this may happen when a woman lies on her back (supine hypotensive syndrome) (Scott, 1968).

    The normal blood volume (in litres) is just under 10 per cent of the body weight (in kilograms). It is not possible to measure it in the circumstances we are considering, and reliance must be placed on clinical signs and on the measurement of operative loss. When it is reduced by more than about 6 per cent, the veins constrict and tachycardia develops. The venous pressure will be low. Later the pulse pressure will fall, followed by the blood pressure as a whole, as the loss reaches about 10 per cent of the blood volume. The appearance of clinical signs will depend in part on the rate of blood loss, which will determine the rate of transfer of interstitial fluid into the intravascular space. Pinching the skin may reveal loss of elasticity and substance. These signs indicate a severe blood volume deficit.

Venous pressure can be measured by examining the neck veins or via a catheter in a central vein. A special unit such as the E-Z Cath is best for this purpose. A 24 inch (60 cm) wide-bore catheter inserted into the median cubital vein at the elbow will have to be advanced almost to its full length to ensure that the tip is in the superior vena cava. It is then connected to a venous manometer set consisting of a 3-way tap, infusion set and 1 metre side arm (drip extension set). The ready-made venous pressure sets (as shown in Figure 2.3) are the most convenient. A centimetre scale is placed on the drip stand, making sure that the zero is at the level of the heart (mid-axillary line in the supine position). If the catheter is properly inserted the level in the side arm should fluctuate both with respiration and with the heart beat. Serial measurements of central venous pressure are a good guide to the state of the blood volume. Venous pressure will be low (-2 to $+1$ cm H_2O) in oligaemia, but will rise to normal (0 to $+5$cm H_2O) with transfusion. Rapid infusion of fluid or the onset of heart failure will lead to an increase of pressure, but it must be remembered that electrolyte solutions are distributed throughout the extracellular fluid and over-infusion may lead to generalised or pulmonary oedema with little or no rise in venous pressure. Artificial respiration, by raising the mean intra-thoracic pressure, will also raise the central venous pressure.

The cardiac output

This is the volume of blood ejected by the heart every minute. The resting value in young adults is as much as seven litres a minute, but it falls to less than five litres a minute in old age. Cardiac output varies with body size and with the metabolic demand for oxygen. For example it rises in fever and thyrotoxicosis. It is high in young children but falls off gradually throughout adult life.

In other words a volume roughly equal to all the blood in the body is circulated once a minute. This volume can rise during exercise to three times the resting level, enabling a much greater quantity of oxygen to be carried to the tissues. In heart disease the response to exercise is usually severely curtailed and even the resting level may be reduced. The response to exercise is an indication of the heart's capacity to respond to any other situation in which an increased cardiac output is called for (e.g. anaemia).

Factors affecting the cardiac output

a)   Contractility of the heart muscle
This is increased by sympathetic stimulation, including sympathomimetic amines, particularly adrenaline, noradrenaline and isoprenaline, and by digitalis. It is also indirectly stimulated by fever, by carbon dioxide

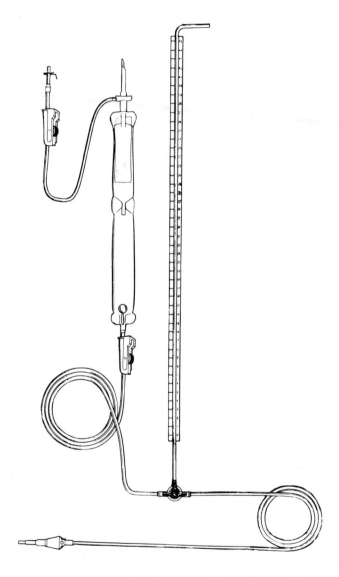

Fig. 2.3   Venous pressure set (Travenol)

retained during under-ventilation of the lungs and in thyrotoxicosis.
Myocardial contractility is reduced by many drugs, including all anaesthetic
agents, although some of these increase sympathetic activity so that the
direct effect on the heart is masked. It is also reduced by many other
factors, particularly be metabolic acidosis (see p. 12), hypoxia, hyperkalaemia, by citrate in transfused blood, by certain infectious agents
(e.g. toxoplasmosis) and in myocarditis due to nutritional deficiency (beri-
beri) or anaemia.

b)   Rhythmicity of the heart
The maximum efficiency of the heart-beat is achieved when the rhythm is
normal. Dysrhythmias reduce the resting level of cardiac output and
severely limit the heart's ability to respond to exercise. For example,
patients with mild disability due to rheumatic heart disease have resting
levels of cardiac output 86 per cent of normal if they are in normal
rhythm, but only 64 per cent if they have atrial fibrillation (Wade and
Bishop, 1962). On exercise the cardiac output in the latter case may be
less than half the normal value. Other types of dysrhythmia, such as
multiple ectopic beats, are also associated with low cardiac outputs.

c)   Venous return
The output of the heart depends largely on the right atrial filling pressure.
When the blood volume is low, the flow of blood back towards the heart
(venous return) is low. Venous tone, controlled by the sympathetic nervous
system, keeps the right atrial pressure constant within limits. Beyond a
certain point the pressure drops: for example, the change from supine to
erect posture is associated with a 20 per cent fall in cardiac output, in spite
of an increase in heart rate. This is because the heart no longer fills to the
same degree and the stroke output falls.

Conversely, distension of the veins with raised central venous pressure
tends to increase cardiac output, but over-distension (due to overinfusion of
fluid or to heart failure) is associated with overfilling of the heart. The
cardiac output falls when this happens.

d)   Heart rate and autonomic control
Changes of cardiac output in response to physiological stimuli are usually
accompanied by changes in heart rate, the stroke volume tending to remain
fairly constant. However, in exceptional situations autonomic factors are
over-riding. An example is seen in oligaemic shock, in which the heart rate
increases because of increased sympathetic activity, but cardiac output
remains low because of the reduced venous return. At rest the heart rate is
influenced by the tone of the vagus (vagal stimulation slows the heart).
Vagal tone is increased as a result of certain reflexes, usually associated with
the stretching of a hollow viscus. Examples important in anaesthesia are
dilating the anal sphincter, pulling on the mesentery and pressing on the

eyes (oculo-cardiac reflex). Sympathetic tone is less important and the
increase in heart rate and contractile force associated with sympatho-
adrenal stimulation is mediated largely by humoral means. Such a response
is elicited by oligaemia, fear and anxiety accompanying illness, hypoxia,
hypercarbia, the stimulus of operation and by certain anaesthetic agents,
particularly ether.

e)   Pathological factors
Fever is accompanied by an increase in cardiac output while hypothermia
has the reverse effect, cardiac output varying with metabolic rate. Hypoxia,
whether acute or chronic, is accompanied by an increase, provided that
circulatory reflexes remain intact. For example, on breathing 12 per cent
oxygen the output increases by 20 per cent. In both these conditions the
increase has the effect of keeping the oxygen flux constant. Marked vasodilation (usually accompanying fever) and arterio-venous fistulae
increase output by increasing venous return. Underventilation of the lungs
leads to a rise in arterial carbon dioxide tension (hypercarbia) which causes
cardiac output to rise (Prys-Roberts, 1967). Anaemia is associated with
reduced blood viscosity, so reducing the resistance to flow through the
capillaries, as a result permitting more rapid flow and quicker return of
blood.

Cardiac output rises during pregnancy to about 50 per cent above the
normal level but returns to the pre-gestation level within two weeks of
delivery. Delivery is accompanied by a redistribution of the blood volume
which in itself causes marked fluctuations of cardiac output. Valvular
disease of the heart, by causing a mechanical obstruction to the flow of
blood, limits the ability of the heart to increase its output in response to
stimulation.

To sum up, the ability of the heart to increase its output in response to
physiological stimuli is limited by any factor which reduces the contractility of the heart, by dysrhythmia, valvular disease, reduction of the
venous return and by all general anaesthetic agents in sufficiently high
doses (see Chapter 3). Moreover, if these factors are severe enough, the
resting level of cardiac output will also be reduced.

Carriage of oxygen in the blood

Oxygen is mainly transported in combination with the haemoglobin of the
blood. One gram of haemoglobin carries 1.34 ml of oxygen and a normal
adult has about 15 grams of haemoglobin per 100 ml of blood. This
volume of blood can therefore carry about 20 ml of oxygen when saturated;
a small quantity of oxygen is also carried in solution in the plasma. In the
lungs oxygen passes from the alveoli to the blood in the pulmonary
capillaries, which becomes saturated. The normal tension of oxygen in
the arterial blood is 100 mg Hg, but the tension in the tissue cells is very

much lower, of the order 5–10 mm Hg. Oxygen passes down this tension gradient from the blood, through the tissue spaces and into the cells. Under resting conditions only about a quarter of the oxygen in the blood will be taken up in this way, and the venous blood returning to the lungs will contain about 15 ml oxygen per 100 ml of blood. In other words, about 25 per cent of the oxygen is extracted from the blood during its passage through the capillaries.

Although the oxygen carrying capacity of a normal subject is about 20 ml per 100 ml, in anaemic patients with low haemoglobin levels the capacity is correspondingly reduced. This reduced capacity is compensated for in two ways. First, a greater proportion of the oxygen is extracted, so reducing the saturation in the venous blood returning to the lungs (see below). This however may lead to appreciable arterial desaturation if intrapulmonary shunting is increased, for example, during artificial respiration under anaesthesia (Marshall and Grange, 1966). Patients with sickle-cell disease may have reduced arterial oxygen tensions (Oduntan, 1969). Secondly, the cardiac output increases mainly as a result of reduced blood viscosity.

The relationship between the degree of saturation of the haemoglobin with oxygen and the oxygen tension is represented by the oxy-haemoglobin dissociation curve (Figure 2.4). The curve is S-shaped, the upper part being almost flat. However the relationship between saturation and tension is not constant, that is to say, the position of the whole curve can change, indicating changes in the affinity of haemoglobin for oxygen. This affinity decreases (i.e. the curve shifts to the right) when oxygen transport is impaired, for example, in anaemia, heart failure, pulmonary insufficiency, at high altitude and in acidaemia (Hjelm et al., 1970). Although a decrease in oxygen affinity may at first sight appear undesirable in these conditions, study of the dissociation curve will show that this is not really so. Because the upper part of the curve is relatively flat, a shift to the right of a few mm Hg makes very little difference to the saturation of the blood leaving the lungs. However, at the capillary level, assuming that the tissue oxygen tension remains the same, the degree of saturation will become much less than normal. That is to say, a much greater proportion, 50 per cent or more, of the oxygen carried in the blood can be extracted by the tissues. This is because the dissociation curve is at its steepest at this level. A decreased affinity for oxygen therefore actually protects the tissues against oxygen starvation.

Fluid and electrolyte balance

Body fluid compartments

Total body water varies with lean body mass and is approximately 60 per cent of body weight. Two thirds is intracellular and one third (equal to

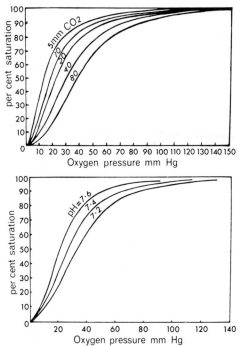

Fig. 2.4 Oxyhaemoglobin dissociation curves, showing the effects of carbon dioxide tension and pH

about 20–25 per cent of body weight) is extracellular. Plasma is only 5 per cent of body weight, the rest of the extracellular fluid (ECF) being interstitial fluid. Addition or loss of water will alter the concentration of electrolytes in the body, while addition or loss of isotonic electrolyte solution will alter the volume of body water.

Salt and water balance

Water intake is normally about 2–2.5 litres per day and is balanced by an equal amount of loss. The loss is of the order of 750 ml in the stools, 1–1.5 litres of urine and 0.5–1.5 litres insensible loss. Catabolism, which follows operation or injury, will release about 0.5–1.5 litres of water per day, but a similar volume of urine will be needed to excrete the other products of catabolism.

Sodium accounts for 90 per cent of the osmotically active cation in the ECF. Intake (as salt) is normally about 55–90 mEq per day (3–5 g). An equal amount is lost, mostly in the urine, but if intake is reduced or salt is lost by other routes, renal output may be less than 20 mEq per day.

Distributional changes

Shifts of fluid between the intracellular and extracellular compartments, or shifts between the interstitial and vascular compartments are termed distributional. They are not necessarily accompanied by changes in the total body water, although in many cases the result is a contraction of ECF volume. Changes in composition can be detected by measuring serum levels, but volume changes can only be detected by clinical signs.

Fluid volume changes due to surgery or trauma

These are very common and are due to losses or gains of isotonic fluids. It is often impossible to say if fluid has moved into the cells, or extravasated into traumatised tissue, atonic bowel, peritoneal exudate or areas of burnt skin. During and after operation the fall in ECF volume due to these losses may amount to several litres in a few hours (Baxter and Shires, 1966). Death is likely to occur when the loss reaches 20 per cent of body weight (10–15 litres in an adult), a volume equivalent to the normal ECF volume (Taylor, 1970). Clinical signs of dehydration appear when the loss is of the order of 2.5 litres and are due largely to reduction in the blood volume. Vasoconstriction, cold, pale, inelastic skin, shrunken tongue, dryness of the mouth and reduced intra-ocular pressure will be followed by tachycardia, oliguria, hypotension and finally clouding of consciousness. The commonest mistake is to underestimate the loss. ECF deficit will be present in many surgical illnesses, particularly intestinal obstruction and obstructed labour. It is the greatest single cause of death in late intestinal obstruction of all types. Hypotension occurring 6–12 hours after operation may also be due to this cause.

Excess ECF volume may result from over-infusion of electrolyte solutions, although this is usually well tolerated, the surplus being excreted by the kidneys. Signs of fluid overload are peripheral oedema and dyspnoea leading to pulmonary oedema. Rise of central venous pressure will only indicate rapid infusion, not a volume excess.

Concentration abnormalities

1)   *Hyponatraemia*

This indicates a relative excess of body water. It occurs when salt-free fluids are given to replace electrolyte loss, when sodium loss is great, or when water intake exceeds water loss. The causes are:

   a) Giving water or salt-poor intravenous fluid to replace electrolyte losses incurred in vomiting, diarrhoea, nasogastric or wound drainage, and the loss of extracellular fluid into the wound, bowel or the cells which occurs in major operations, particularly abdominal operations. Serum levels of sodium and potassium will fall in these circumstances and renal output of these ions will be reduced for a day or two after operation (Shires and Jackson, 1962).

b) Giving water or salt-poor intravenous fluid to patients with increased sodium loss due to other causes. Losses in the urine will increase following the use of diuretics, in some types of renal damage, in some head injuries and in alkalosis. In an unacclimatised subject in a hot environment the sodium loss at rest may exceed 100 mEq per day, although when acclimatisation is complete (after about three weeks) the maximum loss will be about one third of this.

c) Oliguria or anuria due to renal failure, hypotension or urinary obstruction (while water intake is maintained).

d) Decreased insensible loss due to hypothermia or vasoconstriction (in the presence of a normal water intake).

e) Intracellular shift of sodium, which occurs in severe systemic infection.

f) Release of water by catabolism.

Symptoms are rare if the serum sodium is over 120 mEq per litre, but at lower levels headaches and confusion occur, leading occasionally to convulsions or coma, especially in children or old people. A level of less than 100 mEq per litre is extremely rare.

2)   *Hypernatraemia*

In hypernatraemia, the serum sodium level is greater than 150 mEq per litre. This is easily produced when renal function is poor. It indicates a relative water deficiency and is associated with an osmotic gradient between the ECF and the cells, resulting in a reduction of intracellular water. Therefore, when correcting, allowance has to be made for total body water and not just ECF volume. The causes are:

a) Excess renal water loss with inability to excrete sodium. This follows hypoxic damage to the distal tubules and the reduction of ADH secretion caused by some head injuries. Giving hyperosmolar solutions (such as glucose or mannitol) will cause osmotic diuresis. Young infants are unable to excrete sodium efficiently and come into this group.

b) Increased extrarenal water loss occurs in fever (in which insensible loss may reach as much as 3.5 litres per day) and in patients with large granulating areas caused by burns.

c) Excessive salt loading due to infusing hypertonic saline or giving a hyper-osmolar high salt, high protein diet by nasogastric tube. In these cases hypernatraemia may lead to secondary retention of water and even to congestive cardiac failure.

d) Diminished water intake due to starvation, withholding of water during the operative period or inability to swallow.

Symptoms and signs are thirst, which occurs when the deficit is greater

than about 1.5 litres, oliguria with a high urine specific gravity, followed
by the signs of dehydration already mentioned.

3)   *Acid-Base Disturbances*

These may have a profound effect on water and electrolyte balance. Sodium
excretion is greater in alkalosis, which may be the cause of hyponatraemia,
while acidosis reduces it, causing sodium retention. Kidney damage may
prevent the exchange of hydrogen ions for sodium, formation of ammonia
and potassium excretion, leading to metabolic acidosis. Metabolic acidosis
is also due to the anaerobic metabolism which follows tissue hypoxia, to
persistent diarrhoea and to diabetic ketosis. Metabolic alkalosis may be due
to prolonged vomiting and chronic potassium deficiency.

4)   *Potassium balance*

Although the total amount of extracellular potassium is only about 55 mEq,
control of potassium level is extremely important for muscle function,
particularly the function of cardiac muscle. The distribution between the
intracellular and extracellular compartments depends on the acid-base state.
In acidosis hydrogen ions displace potassium from the cells and the plasma
potassium level rises, while the reverse happens in alkalosis. Hyperkalaemia
is due to diminished renal excretion of potassium, extensive tissue
breakdown or underperfusion (especially of the liver), diabetic ketosis or
excessive administration of potassium. It causes confusion, paraesthesiae
and bradycardia, leading to cardiac irregularities, heart block and cardiac
arrest. Hypokalaemia is due to reduced intake in the presence of a normal
rate of excretion (10—20 mEq per day), decreased absorption, diuretics,
diarrhoea, vomiting, increased urinary loss and transfer into the intracellular compartment. Signs are tachycardia leading to cardiac failure, muscle
weakness and hypotonia.

Chapter Three

Pharmacology

Drugs are the anaesthetist's most important tools and a full understanding of their properties is essential for the precise and effective production of anaesthesia. An anaesthetic is seldom a simple matter of giving a single drug, but more often results from the employment of a number of drugs in combination. The actions of a drug will usually be affected by the other drugs and procedures employed. This chapter will endeavour to cover the most important properties of the drugs used in anaesthesia.

Drugs used in premedication

Atropine

Atropine Sulphate B.P. is an alkaloid, being a racemic mixture of d- and l-hyoscyamine. Its principal action is to block transmission of nerve impulses at those post-ganglionic nerve endings at which the transmitter is acetylcholine. It thus blocks the action of the parasympathetic nervous system.

Atropine has little central effect, although it may cause slight drowsiness. It dilates the pupils, but the doses used for premedication do not increase intra-ocular pressure. Bronchial and salivary secretions are reduced by atropine but may become thick and tenacious, while bronchial muscle is relaxed, causing a small increase in deadspace. These effects are very important during anaesthesia with ether, which tends to increase secretions. Sweating (controlled by cholinergic sympathetic fibres) is inhibited and this may occasionally lead to a rise of temperature which can be dangerous in febrile patients.

Small doses of atropine slow the heart, but the usual premedicant doses will cause either no change or a small increase in rate. Used thus, atropine protects against bradycardia due to vagal activity which may occur during operation. However, it may lead to an increased incidence of arrhythmias during induction (Hart and Bryce-Smith, 1963). When tachycardia is already present, atropine causes little further increase in heart rate. Accelerating doses given intravenously may cause multifocal ventricular ectopic beats, but will also increase arterial pressure and cardiac output. After intravenous injection the effect on the heart is immediate, but the effect on secretions develops less rapidly; the increase in cardiac output will only last about half an hour but the effect on heart rate is more prolonged.

Atropine is used in anaesthetic practice to dry secretions and to prevent or treat bradycardia and hypotension which may complicate anaesthesia. The usual dose for premedication is 0.01 mg/kg (see Chapter 5). After intramuscular injection it works in about half an hour, reaching a peak in about one hour. It may be given orally, in which case it acts within about an hour. Intramuscular injection half to one hour before operation is more effective in drying secretions than intravenous injection immediately beforehand. Atropine is partly excreted in the urine but the major part is broken down in the body. It is available in ampoules of 0.5 or 0.6 mg in 1 ml and as tablets containing the same dose.

Hyoscine

Hyoscine Hydrobromide B.P. is a laevorotatory alkaloid. Its actions are similar to atropine, but with some differences. The most important is that hyoscine causes drowsiness and amnesia, while in old people it may lead to excitement and restlessness. It is a more effective drug than atropine for drying salivary and bronchial secretions. It tends to slow the heart rate in normal doses, an effect which may last up to three hours. The usual dose for premedication is 0.01 mg/kg (see Chapter 5). The duration of action is similar to atropine and it may be given intramuscularly or orally.

Diazepam

Diazepam (trade name Valium) is a bendodiazepine which is insoluble in water but freely soluble in organic solvents. It is a potent tranquilliser and anticonvulsant and is highly effective in relieving pre-operative anxiety. Larger doses cause drowsiness and even unconsciousness. It is available as 5 mg and 10 mg tablets, as a syrup (2 mg in 5 ml) and as an injection solution (10 mg in 2 ml). The formation of an abscess after intramuscular injection has been reported. It can be given intravenously. The premedicant dose is 0.25–0.5 mg per kg by mouth two hours before operation, or 0.25 mg per kg intramuscularly one hour beforehand.

Chlordiazepoxide

Chlordiazepoxide hydrochloride B.P. (trade name Librium) was the first benzodiazepine to be introduced. It is similar in action to diazepam but causes little drowsiness. It has the advantage of being water soluble but the intramuscular solution (100 mg in 2 ml) should not be given intravenously. It is also available as 10 mg and 25 mg capsules. The dose used for pre-medication is 2 mg per kg, orally.

Droperidol

Droperidol (trade names Droleptan, Dehydrobenzperidol, Dridol, Inapsin). Droperidol is a 'neuroleptic' drug of the butyrophenone series. It produces a state in which the patient appears sedated and even catatonic, but without any subjective feeling of sedation. Indeed, it may actually induce anxiety (Morrison, Clarke and Dundee, 1970). It makes the patient lie still and quiet, acting as a pharmacological restraining strap. It has adrenergic blocking and anti-emetic effects, but it depresses neither circulation nor respiration, although patients who receive large doses (more than about 20 mg in an adult) may show extra-pyramidal twitching movements and it may aggravate severe depression. It is believed to be mainly metabolised in the liver. Patients who receive droperiodol alone for premedication will obtain no relief of anxiety, and may even experience acute dysphoria.

Droperidol may be used for premedication but only in combination with a true sedative. It reduces the incidence of excitement during induction of ether anaesthesia. It also helps prevent post-operative excitement and vomiting (Crul et al., 1967). It is a valuable aid to the management of patients, such as those having ophthalmic, plastic and ENT operations, who may come to harm from these complications. It is a highly effective drug in the management of excited or semiconscious restless patients, but should not be relied on when restlessness is due to pain.

The dose for premedication is 0.2 mg/kg (10 mg for an adult) by mouth two hours before operation or half this dose by intramuscular injection one hour beforehand. It should *always* be combined with a tranquillising drug such as diazepam (see Chapter 6). For dealing with restless or excited patients 0.1 mg/kg (5 mg in an adult) should be given either intravenously or intramuscularly. For minor procedures and operations under local or regional analgesia droperidol may be combined with an opioid such as morphine or pethidine to help ensure that the patient remains still during the procedure.

Droperidol is available in ampoules containing 10 mg in 2 ml and as 2.5 mg and 10 mg tablets.

Drugs used for the induction of anaesthesia

Thiopentone Sodium B.P.

This is the most commonly used intravenous agent and has a variety of trade names (e.g. Pentothal, Intraval). It is a yellow powder smelling like hydrogen sulphide which dissolves in water to make a strongly alkaline solution, with a pH of 10.8. The 2.5 per cent solution, which is almost isotonic, is now used almost exclusively although the 5 per cent solution is still available but no longer considered safe (see below). It is supplied in 0.5 g ampoules to be dissolved in 20 ml sterile water or in 2.5 g multidose bottles to be dissolved in 100 ml water. The solution is unstable and will become cloudy on keeping: however it will remain useable, particularly if kept in a refrigerator, for several days. For the occasional case, it is better to use an ampoule.

Thiopentone depresses the central nervous system, producing unconsciousness. Cerebral oxygen consumption is reduced and it is an anticonvulsant. It depresses the sympathetic nervous system, but its effect on the para-sympathetic system is not marked. Very small doses produce drowsiness, but also appear to increase sensitivity to pain or discomfort, producing excitement and restlessness. If a large dose is used for unsupplemented anaesthesia, comparatively large incremental doses will be needed. It has been shown that the brain develops 'acute tolerance' to thiopentone and that the blood level at the time of awakening varies with the initial dose (Dundee, 1956), suggesting that there is no advantage to be gained from a large induction dose.

The main effect on respiration is depression but when thiopentone is injected intravenously, apnoea is commonly preceded by yawning or by a series of deep breaths. With normal induction doses apnoea is of very short duration and presents no problems, although transient hiccups may occur. With the larger doses used for unsupplemented anaesthesia for short procedures (see Chapter 7), respiratory depression may need treatment, particularly when the stimulus of operation is no longer present. The cough reflex is not depressed by thiopentone, which prevents it being an ideal introduction to ether, except when followed by a relaxant and endotracheal intubation. Coughing and laryngospasm may occur 'spontaneously' after giving thiopentone, but in fact usually are due to the presence of saliva, mucus or regurgitated stomach contents in the pharynx.

Thiopentone is a powerful cardiovascular depressant, reducing myocardial contractility and causing vaso-dilatation, with a fall in peripheral resistance. After an initial period of depression immediately after intravenous injection, the cardiac output normally increases again and arterial pressure returns to the previous level. It will be dangerous in patients with heart disease, particularly those with myocardial damage, severe valvular disease, pericarditis and complete heart block. Similar risks apply to those with severe toxaemia, hyperkalaemia and metabolic acidosis. These patients have little or no ability to increase cardiac output and as a result become hypotensive after thiopentone. Cardiac arrest may occur in this group.

The rapidity of action of thiopentone is largely determined by the blood flow to the brain (usually about 15 per cent of the cardiac output) and by its fat solubility (oil/water solubility ratio, 4.7). After intravenous injection it circulates rapidly to those tissues, such as the brain, which have a high blood flow. Because the brain has a relatively high lipid content, and because thiopentone passes rapidly through the blood-barrier, the concentration of the drug in the brain rises rapidly (within a few seconds) to equal that in the blood. However, the concentration in the blood begins to fall as the drug passes into other body tissues such as muscle which are less well perfused than the brain. Thiopentone will then pass out of the brain again into the bloodstream and the patient will show signs of awakening. Re-distribution of the drug into the body fat is a slow process because fat is very poorly perfused with blood. Persistently high plasma levels (enough to cause post-operative drowsiness) are only achieved by very large total doses, either in a single injection or by repeated doses.

Thiopentone is almost completely metabolised in the body, mainly by the liver. 10–15 per cent of the drug is broken down each hour, representing a half life of about five hours.

It has been shown that when thiopentone is injected into the bloodstream, crystals of the drug form (Waters, 1966). If the injection has inadvertently been made into an artery these crystals will lodge in peripheral arterioles, blocking the blood supply to the tissues and causing thrombosis of the vessel. Intra-arterial injection is followed by pain the arm or fingers, blanching of the skin and disappearance or weakening of the radial pulse. Gangrene of the fingers may follow. For treatment of this condition see Chapter 7.

Ketamine

This rapidly acting drug produces an anaesthetic state consisting of profound analgesia, normal pharyngo-laryngeal reflexes, mild cardio-vascular stimulation and normal voluntary muscle tone. It is available in an aqueous solution containing 10 or 50 mg per ml. The 10 mg/ml solution is isotonic and is intended for intravenous use, while the 50 mg/ml solution is given by intramuscular injection. The dose is 2 mg/kg by intravenous injection which acts in about 30 seconds and lasts for 5–10 minutes. The intramuscular dose is 10 mg/kg which acts in 3–5 minutes and lasts for 15–30 minutes. It may be used to induce anaesthesia or as the sole anaesthetic agent for minor procedures. Its use is described in Chapter 7.

The principal disadvantages of ketamine is that it causes terrifying hallucinations during the recovery phase. These are sufficiently common to limit its widespread use, although they appear to be almost unknown in young children. It causes increased arterial, intra-ocular and intracranial pressures and is therefore contra-indicated in patients in whom these pressures are already raised. Transient respiratory depression may follow rapid intravenous injection, while nystagmus and clonic movements of the limbs are occasionally seen. Salivation is pronounced during ketamine anaesthesia and atropine or hyoscine are therefore advisable for pre-medication.

Muscle Relaxants

These drugs produce skeletal muscle paralysis by interfering with transmission of the nerve impulse at the neuro-muscular junction. Their chemical
structure is sufficiently like acetyl choline, the physiological transmitter,
for them to become attached to the motor endplates, so preventing acetyl
choline itself combining with the endplate receptors. Because they are less
rapidly removed than acetyl choline they remain on the endplates and
prevent the muscles responding to nerve impulses. Because muscle relaxants
paralyse respiration they should only be used when oxygen and apparatus
for artificial respiration are available.

There are two groups of muscle relaxants. The first, depolarising
relaxants, are so like acetyl choline that they depolarise the muscles and
cause them to contract. After intravenous injection, a wave of fine twitching of the muscles (fasciculation) can be seen passing along the body. The
muscles remain refractory until the drug is hydrolysed by serum cholinesterase, usually within a few minutes. Their action is prolonged in severe
liver disease, in which production of cholinesterase is deficient, when
cholinesterase has been inactivated by anti-cholinesterase drugs or in those
subjects who have a congenital abnormality of the enzyme. The second
group, non-depolarising relaxants, combine at the motor endplates, but do
not cause the muscles to contract nor do they cause fasiculation. They have
a longer duration of action than the commonly used depolarising types
and they are potentiated by ether. Their action can be reversed by giving
an anti-cholinesterase, such as neostigmine, which, by preventing the
breakdown of acetyl choline, increases its concentration at the motor
endplates. Normal transmission of nerve impulses is then restored. The
reversal of non-depolarising relaxants is described at the end of the section
on relaxants in Chapter 8.

Suxethonium Bromide   (*Trade name, Brevedil E.*)

This is a white crystalline powder which is rapidly soluble in water, but the
solution is unstable and should be freshly prepared for each case. The rate
of hydrolysis is greatly increased in an alkaline medium, and it should
therefore not be mixed with thiopentone solution. It is a short acting
depolarising muscle relaxant, its effect normally lasting 2–3 minutes, used
mainly to assist endotracheal intubation, but useful also for short procedures for which profound relaxation is required, such as reduction of a
dislocated hip or shoulder. Because it causes complete paralysis, oxygen
should be given before its use, and artificial respiration performed until
its action wears off. The usual dose is 40 mg, measured as the active cation,
dissolved in 2 ml of water for injection. It is normally given intravenously,
but it is also active after intramuscular injection, although the onset of
the effect is delayed. Its use is described in Chapter 7.

Suxamethonium (*Other names, Succinyl choline, Scoline* (*chloride*), *Brevedil M* (*bromide*), *Anectine*)

This drug is chemically similar to suxethonium and is also a depolarising relaxant, but its duration of action is a little longer, lasting 4—5 minutes. It is used to assist endotracheal intubation and for short procedures which require full muscle relaxation. It is given by the intravenous route, but can also be given intramuscularly.

It is available as the bromide, a white crystalline powder, 40 mg of which is dissolved in 2 ml sterile water. An aqueous solution of the chloride, 100 mg in 2 ml, is also supplied, but the potency of this preparation declines during storage, particularly in the heat and this solution should therefore be stored in a refrigerator. In hot climates the bromide should be used, and should be freshly prepared for each case. Its use is described in Chapter 8.

Both suxethonium and suxamethonium may cause bradycardia, hypotension, and increased bronchial secretions, and their use must be preceded by atropine. In some seriously ill patients, particularly those who have had severe burns, these drugs cause a sharp rise in the plasma potassium level, which may lead to cardiac arrest (Roth and Wüthrich, 1969). Their use should also be avoided in patients in whom the level is already raised (e.g. patients with metabolic acidosis or renal failure). The effect of potassium on the heart can be reversed by giving 100 mg (10 ml of 1 per cent solution) of calcium chloride. Prolonged apnoea occurs in patients whose serum cholinesterase level is severely reduced, necessitating treatment by artificial respiration (see above and Chapter 5). Muscle pains are common after the use of these drugs, particularly in patients who get up and about very soon after operation. Lastly, the intra-ocular pressure rises after suxamethonium and suxethonium, which should not be given to patients with open eye wounds for fear of extruding the ocular contents (Adams and Barnett, 1966). The severity of these complications can be reduced by using a dose no larger than necessary.

Tubocurarine Chloride (*Tubocurarine Chloride, B.P., d-tubocurarine, Tubarine*)

This is a non-depolarising muscle relaxant, derived from South American arrow poison and was introduced into anaesthesia in 1942 by Griffiths and Johnson in Montreal. It is available as a 1 per cent aqueous solution (15 mg in 1.5 ml) and is given intravenously, although it is also absorbed after intramuscular injection. After intravenous injection it acts within 2—3 minutes and lasts 30—40 minutes. About two thirds of any dose is broken down in the body and the rest excreted in the urine. It is used to produce muscle relaxation, particularly for upper abdominal surgery. The usual adult dose for this purpose is 30 mg (0.5 mg/kg) which produces almost complete muscle paralysis. Artificial respiration is therefore essential when tubocurarine is used. The patient is kept asleep with light general anaesthesia until the end of the operation when its action is reversed by neostigmine. This technique is described in Chapter 8.

Tubocurarine has no effect on the heart, but may cause some fall in arterial pressure due to sympathetic ganglion block. Some preparations of curare release histamine and this may both drop the arterial pressure and cause bronchospasm. Tubocurarine is bound to plasma globulins and patients with liver disease, in whom globulin levels are raised, may require very large doses because an unusually high proportion of the dose is so bound (Baraka and Gabali, 1968).

Gallamine Triethiodide B.P.   (Flaxedil)

This is a synthetic non-depolarising relaxant. It is commonly available as a 4 per cent solution (40 mg in 1 ml), but a 2 per cent solution (20 mg in 1 ml) is also made. Its action is similar to tubocurarine, but the effect comes on within 1–1.5 minutes after intravenous injection and lasts 20–30 minutes. The usual adult dose is 80–120 mg (about 1.5 mg/kg) which causes muscle paralysis, so that artificial respiration is essential. It causes tachycardia and may increase cardiac output, so it is suitable for old or very ill patients. Its use may cause increased operative blood loss, particularly in young patients. It is capable of causing ventricular ectopic beats and should not be given to patients who are already receiving halothane, chloroform or trichloroethylene or when tachycardia may be dangerous (as in heart surgery). It is entirely excreted in the urine and should not be given to patients in renal failure. Like tubocurarine it is reversed by neostigmine. Its use is described in Chapter 8.

Pancuronium Bromide   (Pavulon)

This non-depolarising muscle relaxant is an amino-steroid available as an aqueous solution containing 4 mg in a 2 ml ampoule. It is a highly specific neuro-muscular blocking agent, the usual adult dose being 4–6 mg (0.05 mg/kg), which acts for about 45 minutes. It is partially excreted unchanged in the urine. It paralyses respiration, which must be continued artificially, but is reversible by neostigmine. It causes only small increases in heart rate, cardiac output and arterial pressure (Kelman and Kennedy, 1970). It is tending to replace tubocurarine, except where lowering of blood pressure is deliberately sought. The use of pancuronium is described in Chapter 8.

Neostigmine   (trade name Prostigmin)

This drug, which is available as the bromide or the methylsulphate, is an anticholinesterase which inhibits the normal hydrolysis of acetyl choline, so raising its concentration at cholinergic nerve endings. It is used in anaesthesia to reverse the action of the non-depolarising muscle relaxants. Both the muscarinic and nicotinic effects of acetyl choline are enhanced. The muscarinic effects are due to stimulation of post-ganglionic para-sympathetic nerve endings and of sympathetic nerve endings in sweat glands and the uterus. The most important muscarinic effects in anaesthesia are slowing of the heart and hypotension (occasionally accompanied by arrhythmias and cardiac arrest), increase in salivary and bronchial secretions, broncho-constriction, and contraction of hollow viscera. Nicotinic effects are due to stimulation of preganglionic autonomic fibres, the adrenal medulla and of motor nerves to skeletal muscle. It is the last of these effects which is employed when reversing the action of a non-depolarising muscle relaxant. It should be remembered that neostigmine will potentiate depolarising relaxants. Because the muscarinic effects are undesirable, the use of neostigmine must be preceded by atropine, which blocks only the muscarinic effect of acetyl choline. Information about reversal of relaxants is given in Chapter 8.

Inhalational Anaesthetics

Ether   (*Diethyl ether: Anaesthetic ether B.P. and U.S.P.*)

Ether is a colourless, volatile liquid with a characteristic strong pungent smell. It has a molecular weight of 74, boils at 35°C and has a vapour pressure of 442 mm Hg at 20°C. The latent heat of vaporisation is 89 calories per gram. The vapour concentration needed in anaesthesia varies from 2–20 per cent. This means that not only will a high concentration be needed, but that a large amount of heat is required to produce a given concentration. A temperature compensated vaporiser is therefore desirable to prevent a falling off of the concentration as the ether cools. It is flammable in air from 1.85 to 7 per cent and detonable in oxygen above 2 per cent. (Macintosh, Mushin and Epstein, 1963.)

Ether is decomposed by light, heat and by exposure to air, with the formation of peroxide and acetaldehyde which decreases its potency. Decomposition is retarded by copper and by diphemylamine and hydro-quinone, which may be added by the manufacturer. It should be stored in a dark cool place. Peroxides may be detected by adding ml of 10 per cent potassium iodide to 10 ml ether. After shaking and storing for 30 minutes in the dark, their presence will be revealed by a yellow colour in the ether. Aldehydes in ether make Nessler's solution turn yellow or become turbid.

Ether is comparatively water soluble and a high concentration (50–150 mg per 100 ml blood) is needed to achieve anaesthesia. Because it is so water soluble, uptake into the body is not limited by its solubility (which governs the amount that can dissolve in the blood) but by the amount that can reach the alveoli, which is itself determined by the concentration delivered by the vaporiser and by the alveolar ventilation (Chapter 2). Clearly, in order to achieve a quick induction it is desirable to give the patient the highest possible concentration of ether. Haggard (1924) showed that doubling the volume of ventilation halves the induction time. However, the vapour is so irritant that at first a high concentration cannot be breathed without the patient coughing or holding his breath. Once the patient is asleep, the tendency to cough becomes less and up to 20 per cent can be inhaled (see Chapter 7) because the vapour appears to have an inhibitory effect on sensory nerve endings in the upper respiratory tract. Beyond this point the rate of uptake is limited only by the volume of air taken into the alveoli. Fortunately patients who have been properly premedicated show an increase in alveolar ventilation during the later stages of induction and during surgical anaesthesia (Dripps and Severinghaus, 1955; Kubota, Schwizer and Vandam, 1962). On the other hand, if opioids or barbiturates are used for premedication, the alveolar ventilation may be so low that deep anaesthesia is almost impossible to achieve.

Ether is distributed throughout the body in the blood stream and equilibrium between the blood and tissue levels is achieved gradually. The major factor determining the uptake of an anaesthetic by a tissue is the blood flow, the lipoid content of the tissue being rather less important, particularly in the case of ether, whose oil/water solubility ratio is only 3.2 (compared with 330 for halothane). In any case most fatty tissues have a poor blood supply and it takes many hours for them to become saturated with an anaesthetic. The brain, however, not only has a high fat content (12.8 per cent), but its blood flow is greater for its weight than any other tissue in the body. The ether level in the brain will therefore relate closely to the arterial level and if this falls ether will pass out of the brain into the bloodstream again. During induction of anaesthesia, when the tissues are absorbing ether rapidly and the level of ether in the veins is low, the arterial level will vary with the alveolar concentration. This means that changes in the alveolar ventilation (and hence the alveolar ether concentration), due, for example, to breath-holding, have a considerable effect on the depth of anaesthesia. Later on, when the body as a whole is approaching saturation (at the inspired tension), less ether will pass into the tissues and the venous level will be correspondingly higher. Changes in alveolar ventilation will then have less influence on the arterial (and hence the brain) level of ether.

Very little ether is metabolised in the body and 85—90 per cent is excreted in the lungs. Excretion is the reverse of uptake, the rate limiting factor again being the alveolar ventilation. The fall in blood concentration is rapid at first, but elimination from poorly perfused tissues takes several days.

Ether in low concentrations is a powerful analgesic, but it is difficult to take advantage of this property during short procedures because of the difficulty of maintaining an even blood concentration. During an inhalational induction there is often a very marked excitement stage with phonation and movement of the limbs, particularly in young men. As anaesthesia increases in depth this activity lessens, although clonus of the legs is sometimes seen in light surgical anaesthesia. CSF pressure rises, probably due to dilatation of cerebral and meningeal vessels.

Ether causes an increase in salivary secretions which will be severe enough to hinder induction of anaesthesia if atropine or hyoscine is not used before hand. Bronchial muscle is relaxed, but ciliary action is little impaired. Respiration is depressed only in deep surgical anaesthesia.

Ether has a curare-like action, depressing neuro-muscular transmission (Tiers and Artusio, 1960) and potentiating the non-depolarising muscle relaxants. It also depresses spinal reflexes, reducing muscle tone. In light surgical anaesthesia the abdominal muscles contract during expiration, but as anaesthesia deepens the abdominal muscles begin to relax, followed by the intercostal muscles. Beyond this point respiration becomes rapid, shallow and jerky, accompanied by marked tracheal tug and exaggerated movements of the diaphragm. Finally the diaphragm becomes paralysed and respiration ceases. The sympathetic nervous system is stimulated, the level of catecholamines in the blood rising as the concentration of ether in the blood increases (Millar and Morris, 1961). As a result, there is dilatation of the pupils and sweating may occur, while peripheral resistance is maintained by vasoconstriction (McArdle et al., 1968). Other effects are dilatation of coronary arteries and dilatation of the gut with inhibition of its movement. The blood glucose level rises due to mobilisation of liver glycogen, with depletion of the glycogen store. The effect of ether on the heart itself is purely depressant (Etsten and Li, 1960). Deepening anaesthesia is accompanied by a progressive reduction in myocardial contractility and relaxation of vascular tone. However, these effects are normally over-shadowed by intense sympathetic activity which has the overall effect of maintaining or even increasing cardiac output and arterial pressure (Kubota, Schweizer and Vandam, 1962; Jones, et al., 1962; Gregory et al., 1971). In deep surgical anaesthesia, the heart rate begins to slow again and arterial pressure may fall. This suggests that the direct cardiovascular effects of ether are beginning to predominate over the sympathetic nervous system effect. The sympathetic effect will be abolished by high spinal block, by ganglionic blocking drugs, by alpha adrenergic blocking agents (including anti-hypertensive drugs) and by reserpine, but probably not by metabolic acidosis (Sodipo, personal communication). A patient taking a beta-adrenergic blocking drug is also likely to be at risk from an ether anaesthetic. This type of drug blocks the beta effects of sympathetic stimulation, particularly the effects on the heart and on metabolism and injection into a patient receiving ether will therefore cause a sudden marked fall in arterial pressure. The effect of sympathetic stimulation is abolished and the heart is exposed to the direct effect of the ether, which causes bradycardia and even cardiac arrest (Jorfeldt et al., 1966).

Temporary depression of renal and hepatic function occurs in normal patients. Infants and patients with cirrhosis may develop metabolic acidosis due to failure of the liver to metabolise lactic acid. The latter may also suffer harm from the depletion of liver glycogen. Well conducted anaesthesia in normal subjects does not cause metabolic acidosis (Beecher, Francis and Afinson, 1950). The uterus is relaxed. Ether crosses to the foetus so that prolonged anaesthesia may depress it. Vomiting is no commoner after a properly conducted ether anaesthesia than with any other agent (Holmes, 1965; Mehta et al., 1969), but prolonged deep anaesthesia (which is not recommended) is associated with vomiting.

The clinical use of ether is described in Chapters 7 and 8.

Halothane   (trade name Fluothane)

Halothane is a heavy (M.W. 197), colourless liquid with a characteristic sweetish smell. It boils at 50°C and has a vapour pressure of 241 mm Hg at 20°C. The latent heat of vaporisation is 39 calories per gram and as the effective anaesthetic concentration is between 0.5 and 2 per cent, cooling of the vaporiser is not a problem. However, because of its potency, it is easy to give an overdose and an accurately calibrated vaporiser is essential. Halothane is much less water soluble than ether, its oil/water solubility coefficient being 330. There is little difficulty in achieving an adequate alveolar concentration and the cardiac output is as important as the alveolar ventilation in determining its rate of uptake from the lungs.

Halothane can produce deep surgical anaesthesia with little excitement during induction, which is quicker than with ether. It does not stimulate breathing at any stage and during surgical anaesthesia respiration becomes more shallow than normal, with a fall in alveolar ventilation and a rise in carbon dioxide tension. It is thus unsuitable as a sole anaesthetic with air alone (Bryce-Smith and O'Brien, 1956), so an oxygen-rich mixture should be used because of the risk of hypoxia. An advantage is that it is not irritant to the larynx and does not stimulate secretions.

Halothane does not have the same muscle relaxing effect as ether. It depresses myocardial contracility and sensitises the heart to injected adrenaline with the risk of ventricular fibrillation. A raised carbon dioxide level will also lead to the appearance of extrasystoles during halothane anaesthesia. Bradycardia and hypotension are common and can be treated by small intravenous doses of atropine (0.25–0.3 mg), but larger doses may cause extrasystoles and should be avoided. Halothane causes vaso-dilatation, the overall effect on the circulation being like that of sympathetic nervous system paralysis.

Halothane has no effect on renal function. It is not directly hepatotoxic, but sensitivity to repeated administrations occurs very rarely. Profound uterine relaxation is produced and it is not suitable for operative deliveries because of the risk of post-partem bleeding. Most of the drug is excreted unchanged, only a small proportion being metabolised in the liver.

Trichloroethylene   (*trade name Trilene*)

Trichloroethylene is a liquid of molecular weight 131. It boils at $87°C$, has a vapour pressure of 58 mm Hg (at $20°C$) and is highly lipoid soluble with an oil: water solubility coefficient of 400. Its latent heat of vaporisation is 58 calories per gram. It is coloured with Waxoline Blue dye for identification purposes. It has a characteristic smell and is non-explosive.

Trichloroethylene is a powerful analgesic, but a weak general anaesthetic. Attempts to produce deep anaesthesia lead to the development of rapid, shallow breathing with carbon dioxide retention and cardiac arrhythmias. The drug is partially broken down in the liver, mainly to trichloracetic acid, but the majority is excreted unchanged.

Trichloroethylene can be used in the Oxford Miniature Vaporizer to provide analgesia in concentration between 0.5 and 1 per cent. This is valuable in obstretics, for painful dressings, changes of plaster and similar operations. It may also be used in combination with halothane, its analgesic effect complementing the strong narcotic action of halothane (see Chapter 8). Its use in the Bryce-Smith Induction Unit for assisting induction of ether anaesthesia in children is described in Chapter 10. It may also be used to maintain unconsciousness in patients who have been given relaxants and artificial respiration (see Chapter 8).

Chloroform B.P.

This is a clear, sweet-smelling liquid, with a molecular weight of 199. It is lipoid soluble (oil:water solubility coefficient 100). It is non-inflammable but exposure to an open flame or spark leads to the formation of phosgene. The boiling point is $61°C$, the vapour pressure at $20°C$ is 160 mm Hg and the latent heat of vaporisation 67 calories per gram.

Chloroform is a powerful anaesthetic agent. It depresses the myocardium and peripheral vascular tone, leading to a fall in arterial pressure. Cardiac arrhythmias are common and cardiac arrest, due to ventricular fibrillation or to asystole, is a well recognised danger, particularly during induction of anaesthesia. Bradycardia is common, but is prevented by atropine. Asystole is usually due to overdosage, but may be attributed to vagal inhibition of the heart. It is a powerful respiratory depressant, leading to anoxia and carbon dioxide retention, unless respiration is assisted. It is hepatotoxic, particularly in poorly nourished patients.

In spite of these disadvantages it is still widely employed. If used with care from a calibrated vaporiser, the danger of giving chloroform may not be prohibitive (Bhalla et al., 1967; Oduntan, 1968). Concentrations of up to 2 per cent are needed for induction. When halothane is not available, it can be used in the Bryce-Smith Induction Unit or the O.M.V. to assist the induction of ether anaesthesia. It should be remembered that the cost of 3 ml of halothane (the normal induction dose) is only 5p.

Drugs used for post-operative analgesia

The use of analgesics is discussed in Chapter 9. These drugs are collectively known as 'opioids', meaning any natural or synthetic drug that has morphine-like pharmacological actions (Jaffe, 1970).

Morphine Sulphate B.P.

This opium alkaloid is still the standard by which other strong analgesics are judged. It relieves pain and usually produces euphoria and sleepiness. It depresses respiration, producing, slow, deep breathing, it abolishes the cough reflex and reduces the normal ventilatory response to physiological stimulus such as a raised carbon dioxide level. It constricts the pupil and gut sphincters and frequently causes vomiting. It may lower blood pressure and cause bradycardia and postural hypotension. It is addictive. The usual dose is about 0.2 mg per kg given by intramuscular injection. The effect will last 2–3 hours.

Pethidine Hydrochloride B.P.   (Other names, Meperidine hydrochloride U.S.P., Dolantin, Dolosal, Isonipecaine, Pantalgin)

Pethidine is a commonly used synthetic morphine-like analgesic. It has a shorter duration of action than morphine and causes less euphoria and sleepiness. It depresses respiration in the same way as morphine, but unlike morphine it tends to relax smooth muscle. It may cause hypotension, nausea and vomiting. It is approximately one tenth as powerful as morphine and is given in a dose of about 1 mg per kg. It is addictive.

Pethidine may cause prolonged coma, restlessness or convulsions and even death in patients receiving monoamine oxidase inhibitors. About 80 per cent of the drug is normally degraded in the liver. Monoamine oxidase inhibitors are thought to inhibit the enzymes responsible for this process. See also Chapter 6.

Pentazocine   (other names, Fortral, Talwin)

This is a synthetic analgesic which has similar pain-relieving and respiratory depressant properties to other opioids. However, it lacks their sedative and euphoriant effect and is regarded as non-addictive. For this reason it is not subject to dangerous drug controls, which make it less of a temptation to thieves and simplifies stock control. It causes little nausea, vomiting or constipation, making it a good drug for post-operative use. Unlike opioids, respiratory depression due to pentazocine is not reversed by nalorphine. It can be treated with methylphenidate (ritalin) 0.5 mg per kg intravenously (Telford and Keats, 1965). The usual adult dose is 60 mg (about 1 mg per kg), by intramuscular injection.

Nalorphine Hydrobromide B.P. (*other names, Lethidrone, Nalline*)

This drug is n-allyl-normorphine and is closely related chemically to morphine. It acts as an antagonist to most morphine-like drugs in the usual dose, which is 5—10 mg for an adult (0.1mg/kg), but very large doses may themselves depress respiration. Not only will it antagonise the respiratory depressant effects of opioids, but it will also antagonise all other effects, including the analgesic effect. It is not effective against pentazocine, itself an opioid antagonist.

Local anaesthetics

Lignocaine (*Xylocaine, Xylotox, Lidocaine, Duncaine*)

A very stable local anaesthetic with a quick onset of action and a duration of 1—2 hours. 1 per cent solution is sufficient for sensory nerve block, while 2 per cent is needed to block motor nerves and for topical analgesia. 5 per cent water-miscible paste may be used for lubricating endotracheal tubes, reducing the incidence of post-intubation coughing. The maximum safe dose is 3 mg/kg (about 200 mg for an adult man). Its rate of absorption can be reduced by adding adrenaline (ideally 1: 250 000) which permits the maximum dose to be raised to 7 mg/kg. An aerosol which delivers 10 mg lignocaine per puff is very useful for spraying the larynx before intubation. This is of particular value in children, in whom it is very easy to give an overdose of topical lignocaine. The toxic effects are cardiac depression, drowsiness, unconsciousness and convulsions. They are treated by giving the patient 100 per cent oxygen to breathe. Convulsions are managed by giving a short-acting muscle relaxant and ventilating the patient artificially until they disappear. Thiopentone will also control the convulsions, but only at the expense of further cardiac depression. Diazepam (5—10 mg intravenously) will also control convulsions but may cause respiratory depression.

Bupivicaine (*Marcaine*)

This is a very powerful and long-acting local anaesthetic, with a quick onset of action and duration of 8—10 hours. 0.5 per cent solution is suitable for motor nerve block, while a sensory block can be achieved by 0.25 per cent solution. The safe dose is 2 mg per kg. It is very useful for intercostal block in abdominal surgery (described in Chapter 8). The advantage is that the block lasts for up to ten hours providing valuable analgesia of the anterior abdominal wall in the post-operative period and thus reducing the need for opioids.

Cinchocaine   (*Nupercaine*)

This is also a very powerful drug which acts for about three hours but is considered too toxic for infiltration anaesthesia. However, it has held its place for spinal (subarachnoid) block. For this pupose a 0.5 per cent (1:200) solution containing 6 per cent glucose, which makes it hyperbaric, is used. This solution will withstand repeated autoclaving for 30 minutes at 115°C or 10 pounds pressure, and although this will make it turn brown due to caramelisation of the glucose, it will still remain fairly effective.

Procaine

Procaine was the first synthetic local anaesthetic but is now considered too toxic for infiltration anaesthesia. It is still an extremely useful drug for producing spinal (subarachnoid) block largely because its duration of action is only about one hour. As the majority of operations performed under spinal anaesthesia take less than this time, the possibility of post-operative complications due to persistent anaesthesia, such as hypotension, is avoided. Ampoules containing 100 mg dry crystals are recommended. These are dissolved in 2 ml cerebrospinal fluid to make a 5 per cent solution, which is hyperbaric. Solutions stronger than 5 per cent may cause nerve damage.

Table 3.1   Approximate prices in Great Britain of the drugs recommended

	pence
Atropine (0.5 mg ampoule)	0.5
Atropine (0.5 mg tablets)	0.5
Bupivicaine 0.5% (10 ml ampoule)	17.0
Chlordiazepoxide (25 mg tablets)	2.0
Chlordiazepoxide (100 mg ampoule)	18.0
Cinchocaine 1:200 (2 ml ampoule)	20.0
Diazepam (10 mg ampoule)	9.0
Diazepam (10 mg tablets)	1.8
Droperidol (10 mg ampoule)	22.0
Droperidol (10 mg tablets)	3.5
Ether 250 ml	5.5
Gallamine (80 mg ampoule)	6.4
Halothane 250 ml	413.0
Hyoscine (0.4 mg ampoule)	2.0
Hyoscine (0.4 mg tablets)	0.1
Ketamine (10 ml ampoule)	146.0
Lignocaine 1% (20 ml ampoule)	4.5
Morphine (10 mg ampoule)	1.3
Pancuronium (4 mg ampoule)	10.0
Pethidine (100 mg ampoule)	1.0
Pentazocine (60 mg ampoule)	19.7
Procaine	7.4
Suxamethonium bromide (40 mg ampoule)	7.4
Suxamethonium chloride (100 mg ampoule)	3.6
Suxethonium bromide (100 mg ampoule)	8.0
Tubocurarine (15 mg ampoule)	9.0
Thiopentone (0.5 mg ampoule)	10.0
Trichloroethylene 250 ml	16.5

Chapter Four

Apparatus

The E.M.O. system consists of vaporisers for volatile anaesthetics, used either alone or in series, together with valves, bellows or self-inflating bags for artificial respiration, and accessories. Although these items were originally introduced at different times and often for different purposes, they form a modular system which can be assembled in various ways to suit different requirements. The possible combinations are discussed in Chapter 6.

The E.M.O. Inhaler   (*Epstein and Macintosh, 1956*)

The E.M.O. (Fig.4.1) is 23 cm in diameter and 24 cm high and weighs 6.5 kg with the water compartment full. A cross-section is shown in Figure 4.2. It has an annular ether vaporising chamber (V), lined with wicks. Surrounding this is a water compartment (W) which acts as a heat capacity. This, in conjunction with an automatic thermocompensating valve (T), prevents any rapid fall of temperature even when high concentrations are delivered. The indicated concentration remains effectively constant over a wide range of respiration frequencies and tidal volumes. This is achieved by a carefully determined relationship between the volumes of the various chambers and the flow directed through them by bell-mouthed and sharp-edged orifices. It was designed for draw-over use in which flow is created by suction (the patient's inspiratory effort) at the outlet, rather than by applying pressure at the inlet, and the air passages are relatively large, offering a low resistance to breathing. The air inlet of the inhaler communicates with a large chamber with two outlets. One of these gives access to the main ether chamber via the closing mechanism. This device seals off the entry to the ether chamber when the control indicator is in the 'Transit' position (to prevent the ether being spilled). Also incorporated in the closing mechanism is an inlet relief valve which allows air to enter the inhaler if the main air inlet becomes blocked. The other outlet port leads into the small chamber in the centre of the control rotor beneath the concentration indicator. This is fully open in the 'Transit' position but as the concentration indicator is moved around towards the 20 per cent position, it

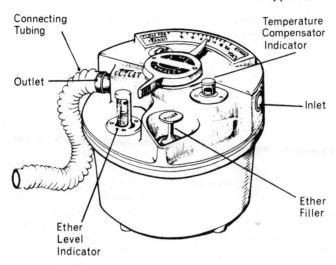

Connecting Tubing

Outlet

Temperature Compensator Indicator

Inlet

Ether Filler

Ether Level Indicator

Fig. 4.1 General view of the E.M.O. inhaler

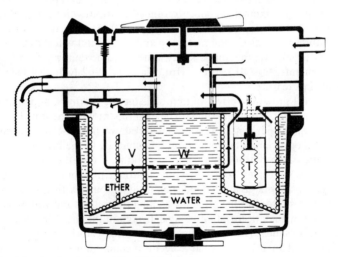

Fig. 4.2 Sectional view of the E.M.O. inhaler

closes progressively, so directing a greater proportion of the air into the ether chamber.

The central chamber beneath the concentration indicator has a second inlet port leading from the ether vaporising chamber via the thermo-compensating valve. This port is fully closed in the 'transit' position but opens progressively as the indicator is moved towards the 20 per cent position, permitting extra air to leave the vaporising chamber. The outlet port from the central chamber gives permanent access to the main inhaler outlet.

The control mechanism thus directs a progressively larger proportion of the air through the ether chamber without altering the total flow through the inhaler. It also seals the ether chamber when the inhaler is not in use.

The temperature compensating thermostat allows more air to pass through the vaporising chamber when the ether gets colder. It is effective in holding the concentration constant between 15° and 30°C. It also adjusts automatically for changes in barometric pressure, such as the reduction occurring at high altitudes (Ghose, 1964). The active element is a sealed capsule containing liquid ether. Ether not only has the correct coefficient of expansion, but in the event of leakage, no harm will follow. The capsule will of course continue to operate with changes of ambient temperature even when the inhaler is not in use. It should normally last about ten years, but eventually the continuous flexing of the bellows will lead to failure from metal fatigue.

There is an indicator on the compensating unit which shows red if the temperature is too high (over 32°C). If this happens, the vaporizer will no longer deliver the indicated concentration (the output will be high at the lower end of the scale, but low at the upper end). At normal working temperatures (20–25°C), the metal top and black band will show. If only the metal top shows, the unit is faulty and should be removed for repair or replacement. Mark III E.M.O.'s (from January 1962 to June 1964) do not have this feature.

Figure 4.3 shows the effect of immobilising the thermo-compensator in the 20°C position (Epstein, 1958). The experiment was performed with the pointer set at 12 per cent. The solid line (B) shows how the concentration varied with environmental temperature, in contrast to the broken line (A) obtained with the thermo-compensator working. If the ether in the chamber becomes too hot (after storage in a hot environment), some ether must be vaporised by opening the filler and sucking air through with the bellows for a few minutes. This has the effect of cooling the inhaler and will prevent a dangerously high concentration being delivered in the first few breaths. As ether vaporises, heat is consumed at the rate of 89 calories per gram of liquid, more than any other volatile agent in common use. Because ether is also used in higher concentration than other agents, efficient temperature control is essential.

All models of the E.M.O. and its accessories are designed so that the outlet connections (towards the patient) are male tapers and the inlet connections female. Early models have the old facemask size tapers (23.6 mm cone), but since January 1966 the British Standard (B.S. 3849: 22 mm cone) tapers have been fitted. Adapters are available to join together items with different sized tapers, although in some cases it may

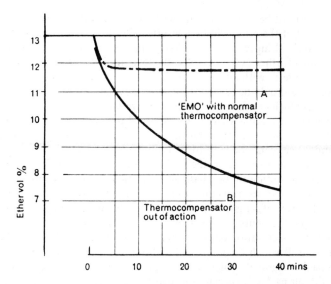

Fig. 4.3   Graphs showing how the concentrations delivered by the E.M.O. depend on the action of the thermo compensator. The control lever was set at '12' while air was blown through by a sine-wave pump at 22 breaths per minute and a minute volume of 9 litres

be found more convenient to use a short length of corrugated tubing instead.

When supplied the water jacket is dry and must be filled with approximately 1200 ml of cold distilled water. To fill the water jacket the inhaler is inverted and the filler unscrewed (older models have a coin slot). Mark I E.M.O.'s (manufactured before June 1960, serial nos. 1—2859) have aluminium water jackets and the water level must be checked every three months because chemical action may lead to the generation of gas which may damage other parts of the inhaler. Mark II, Mark III and Mark IV E.M.O.'s have stainless steel jackets and need only a yearly water level check. In freezing conditions, automobile antifreeze solution containing 25 per cent glycol should be used.

When filling with ether, the control must be turned to the zero position at the bottom on the scale rather than to the 'Transit' position so that air can escape from the vaporising chamber as the ether is poured in. The filler must be held down during filling; it springs back automatically afterwards. Mark I inhalers have fillers which must be lifted and turned. This type may be left open by mistake so that extra air enters the chamber and vaporises too much ether, delivering a very high concentration to the patient. There is a level gauge consisting of a float and indicator. The inhaler must not be overfilled otherwise the wicks will be covered and vaporisation of the ether will be prevented (Prior, 1964). It takes 150 ml to fill it to the 'Empty' mark (this being the amount soaked up by the wicks) and a further 300 ml to raise the level to 'Full'. If it becomes necessary to refill with ether during the course of an anaesthetic, the control knob should be turned to the zero position. otherwise a dangerously high concentration will be delivered.

The concentration is selected by a control pointer which is moved along a scale marked at 1 per cent intervals up to 10 per cent, and then at 15 per cent and 20 per cent concentrations (volume to volume).

Being a draw-over inhaler, the E.M.O. is designed to work with flows which vary according to the phase of respiration. Figure 4.4 shows how the concentration remains constant at different minute volumes (Epstein, 1958). However, if air is blown through the inhaler, either with a self-inflating bag (Clementsen, 1963), or by an automatic ventilator (Millar, 1964), the concentration delivered may be greater than indicated. This is because the air which is compressed within the inhaler during inspiration passes back towards the inlet during expiration. When the next breath is given, this air passes once again through the ether chamber, picking up extra ether vapour. On the other hand, when the E.M.O. is used with a constant flow of gas (as in paediatric practice), the concentration delivered is somewhat less than indicated (Epstein, H. G., personal communication). Table 4.1 shows how the concentration varies with three different continuous flows. This doesn't represent a serious problem in clinical use if the flow is greater than 10 litres a minute. The E.M.O. has a very low resistance to flow (less than 1.25 cm H_2O at 40 litres/min).

Apart from physical damage or misuse (such as putting in volatile agents other than ether or using phenol type antiseptics), an E.M.O. should require no maintenance for five years. In hot, humid climates the air drawn

Table 4.1　Percentage concentrations delivered by the E.M.O. inhaler at three different continuous flows. Measurements made at 20° C. (Figures kindly supplied by Dr. H. G. Epstein.)

		Control setting (per cent)					
		2	3	4	6	10	15
Flow (l/min)	7	1.2	1.9	2.5	4.2	7.4	11.8
	9	1.5	2.5	3.5	5.4	9.0	11.8
	11	1.6	2.7	3.9	5.6	9.0	10.7

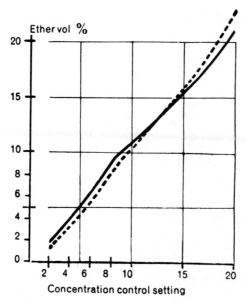

Fig. 4.4 Graph showing that the concentrations delivered by the E.M.O. are unaffected by the minute volume. The solid line represents a minute volume of 8.5 litres and the dotted line 3.5 litres, the respiration rate delivered by the sine-wave pump remaining constant at 20 breaths a minute. Temperature 24°C

into the inhaler will deposit water in the cold ether chamber. This will eventually dilute the ether, limiting the efficiency of the system. Under such conditions the E.M.O. should be drained at the end of every day. Simple checks of the moving parts can be made by the user. The main fault likely to develop on earlier models is that the control pointer may stick (Stetson, 1968). This is most likely to occur if an inhaler is left for long periods full of ether without being used. It may also follow the use of ether dispensed from lacquered cans. The lacquer becomes dissolved in the ether during filling and is deposited in the E.M.O. when the ether subsequently evaporates. Use of trichloroethylene or halothane, apart from corroding the metal of the interior, will also lead to the deposition of gummy material on the rotor, causing it to stick. If the unit is going to be stored for any length of time, drain the ether chamber and open the control fully to allow all the vapour to escape, otherwise oxidation of the ether will occur. The latest version (Mark IV, serial nos. 8894 onwards, made since 1971) has a modified rotor which eliminates this difficulty. Stetson also warns that dust may work into the rotor, making its action stiff. This complication can be avoided by always using a dust filter on the air inlet.

The following checks should be carried out on the inhaler every three months:

1) The level indicator is checked by inverting the inhaler (with the concentration control at 'Transit'), when it should fall freely to the 'Full' position. When refilling check that the quantity of ether poured in agrees roughly with the figures given above.

2) Connect the bellows to the inlet of the E.M.O. and block the outlet. While the control knob is turned to the 'Transit' position and the filler held open, the bellows are compressed; no air should escape through either the top of the closing mechanism or through the filler. This tests that the control rotor and closing mechanism are airtight.

3) When the filler is released and the control pointer turned to 10 per cent this is repeated to check that the filler is not leaking.

4) The bellows is then attached to the outlet and while the E.M.O. air inlet is blocked (and the bellows outlet blocked in the case of the P.B.U.), the control knob is set at '2' and an attempt is made to suck air through the safety release valve. If the valve is working correctly, air can be heard hissing through.

Unit construction and standardisation of parts enable the user to exchange main components himself. Stocks of spares and service facilities are available on a service exchange basis from distributors. When ordering spares from the manufacturer or distributor, the serial number of the inhaler should *always* be given. However, the following notes on dismantling may help in cases of difficulty:

1) The level indicator is retained by three screws round the base which should be completely removed. The indicator will then lift out vertically.

2) The closing mechanism and safety valve has three screws. To remove this unit the two diagonally opposed clamping screws, marked 'A' in Figure 4.5 should be slackened by two or three turns. It can then be lifted out completely. When properly adjusted, the concentration indicator should depress the domed head of the closing mechanism without due force. An adjustment screw ('B') is provided.

3) The filler is screwed into a threaded flange in the main casting. A special screwdriver is needed to engage the slots in the filler, but it is most unlikely ever to need replacing.

4) The temperature compensating unit has three screws which should be loosened by 3 to 5 turns and then pushed down until their heads are level with the surface. It should then lift out completely, but in a much used inhaler the sealing gaskets may stick. In this case the screws should be further slackened and the unit rocked gently in order to release it. New seals should always be fitted when assembling again (see the manufacturer's instruction book). After removing the unit, place the canister part in iced water for a couple of minutes. Then, with the finger and thumb round the lower sealing ring, press the stepped valve disc upwards (against a strong

Table 4.2. Summary of possible faults in the E.M.O. inhaler.

Fault	Cause	Remedy
Ether escaping (in 'Transit' position)	a) Broken level indicator glass	Replace level indicator
	b) Broken indicator glass on temperature compensator	Replace temperature compensator unit (Mk I and II only)
	c) Closing mechanism not shutting	Replace closing mechanism unit
Concentration high but falling off rapidly	a) Temperature compensator not operative	Check unit, replace if necessary
	b) Filler left open (Mk. I only)	Close filler
Concentration too low	a) Leak in circuit	Check for leaks, rectify
	b) Relief valve on closing mechanism stuck	Test (4) above, replace unit or fit new washer
	c) Temperature compensator not working	Check unit, replace if necessary
	d) Overfilled with ether	Pour out excess
Level indicator fails to rise	a) Broken float – moves on inversion but not when ether is added	Fit new unit
	b) Float caught by frayed wick	Remove unit and cut away surplus wick
	c) Caught by collapsed ether compartment due to gas build-up in water jacket (Mk. I only)	Return to makers or service agent
Rotor seized	a) Use of ether from lacquered cans or of unsuitable agent	Empty ether, stand in hot water, apply penetrating oil, attempt to free
	b) Storage for long periods without emptying	Return to makers or service agent

spring) and downwards (weaker spring). If the disc has become stuck on its spindle, this should free it, but if it cannot be freed the whole unit must be replaced. If it can be freed, move it up and down several times to make sure it moves easily. Then replace the canister in iced water to see that the disc moves down and the visual indicator falls. When the unit is transferred to warm water ($40°C$), the disc and indicator should rise until the disc

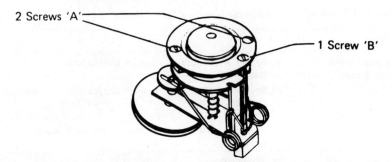

Fig. 4.5   The closing mechanism and safety valve of the E.M.O. The two clamping screws are marked 'A', while screw 'B' is used for adjustment

completely blocks the hole in the lower sealing ring. Dry the unit before replacing it. *Never* unscrew the nuts at the top of the stem or the grub screw at the top of the can.

5) The rotor may become stiff or seize solid. The inhaler should then be emptied of ether and a little penetrating oil or paraffin (kerosene) applied around the control pointer. Gentle warmth (standing in hot water), will help, but it may take several hours to release the joint. The lever should be worked gently to and fro, but no undue force should be applied. If this doesn't work the inhaler should be returned to the makers.

6) The inhaler will not normally need to be sterilised because it is protected from the patient by the non-return valves. In case of external contamination, it should be washed with soap and water followed by ether. Full sterilisation should only be carried out with ethylene oxide gas.

The Oxford Miniature Vaporiser (O.M.V.)

This small vaporiser was designed by Macintosh and Epstein of Oxford (Parkhouse, 1966). It is a simple, portable inhaler capable of delivering fairly accurate concentrations within defined limits, over short periods. It is designed for less volatile agents than ether, such as halothane, methoxy-flurane and trichloroethylene. In particular it is meant as an induction unit for use with the E.M.O., when it should be plugged into the outlet of the latter. It should never be fitted to the inlet of the E.M.O., otherwise halothane will be drawn in, causing corrosion. It can be used with a continuous gas flow for supplementation of relaxant anaesthesia. When combined with an inflating device it can be used as a draw-over anaesthetic apparatus on its own to provide anaesthesia or analgesia (Boulton, 1966, Prior, 1972).

Figure 4.6 shows the general appearance of the vaporiser which is

Table 4.3. Serial numbers and identifying features of different marks of E.M.O.

Mark	Date	Serial numbers	Modifications
I	Before June 1960	1000—2859	Aluminium water jacket, pull up filler
II	June 1960—December 1969	2860—8893	Stainless steel water jacket, push-down filler
III	January 1962—June 1964	Between* 3,500—4,500	No visible temperature indicator
IV	October 1971 onwards	8894 onward	PTFE coated control rotor

* About 400 Mark III inhalers were made, concurrently with the Mark II model

13.5 cm high and weighs 1060 g (with the water jacket full). A control pointer moves across a scale which gives volumetric percentage concentrations at 25°C ambient temperature. There will be small deviations from the indicated concentrations with time and temperature. Figure 4.7 shows this effect when the O.M.V. is used for halothane. The output is never greater than indicated and is unaffected by positive pressure, so it is safe to place it on the patient's side of the bellows (Parkhouse, 1966).

Alternative scales for halothane (HAL 0—4 per cent) inethoxyflurane (MOF 0—0.6 per cent) and trichloroethylene (TCE 0—1.5 per cent) are

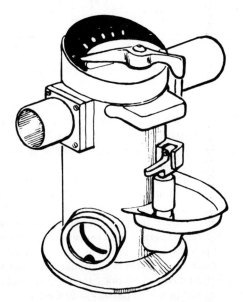

Fig. 4.6   General view of the Oxford Miniature Vaporiser (O.M.V.)

available. Table 4.4 shows how these scales compare. The base contains a water jacket which acts as a heat source. Under freezing conditions there is a danger of rupturing the jacket, which is therefore filled with 25 per cent glycol automobile antifreeze at the factory. When used with the E.M.O., the flow of gas through the vaporiser should be from right to left

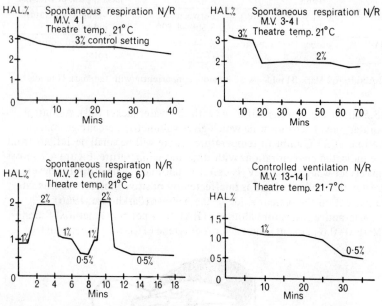

Fig. 4.7   Graphs showing how the concentrations delivered by the O.M.V. correspond with the control settings under different conditions of use

(when looking at the front). Note that there is another version designed for gas machines in which the gas flows from left to right. The direction of flow is marked by an arrow on units made after April 1968 (serial nos. 58–1 onwards). A choice of B.S. 3849 or old facemask inlet and outlet tapers is available.

The O.M.V. has a special filler designed to limit the volume of anaesthetic used. This useful economy device is operated by a lever which must be pressed fully down to open the filling port. There are two springs in the mechanism so that the initial movement of the lever, which opens an air relief valve, is effected against light pressure and heavier pressure must be applied to open the actual filler. The built-in funnel surrounding the filler contains about 10 ml which is convenient for most induction purposes. It is enough to cover about one eighth of the level indicator. A second 10 ml dose may be added initially if desired, but no more. The indicator is designed so that some liquid remains in the chamber even

when it can no longer be seen in the window. During continuous use it
is usual to add more liquid when this happens. The control should be
turned to the zero position when re-filling. Unused liquid can be drained
back into the bottle by pressing the filler level right down and tipping
the vaporiser.

Table 4.4. Conversion scales for the O.M.V.

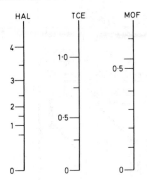

A cross-section of the vaporiser is shown in Figure 4.8. The wicks are
made of stainless steel gauze which will not be corroded by any anaesthetic
in current use. Prolonged use with halothane or trichloroethylene will
make the control slider stick, due to accumulation of their waxy additives.
These can be washed out with alcohol (e.g. methylated spirit) or ether.
The inlet is stopped up with a rubber bung and the vaporiser turned on
its side. The control pointer is moved from side to side while the cleaning
fluid is poured in through the outlet port. The vaporiser should be completely filled and allowed to stand for five minutes before emptying. The
vapour of the cleaning fluid should then be removed by opening the
control fully and blowing air through the vaporiser for 10—15 minutes
with the inflating bellows.

The water jacket is filled at the factory and usually needs no attention.
In hot climates some leakage may occur. To top up the water jacket the
filler on the bottom is unscrewed with a screwdriver and water added with
a syringe and needle. The makers suggest that both these points are
attended to every three months. No other servicing is normally needed.

Bryce-Smith Induction Unit

This is designed to facilitate induction of ether anaesthesia with halothane
(Bryce-Smith, 1964). It is smaller and simpler than the O.M.V., weighing
450 g. It consists of a chamber (5.7 cm in diameter and 12 cm long) containing a large baffle which deflects the air down onto the wick, as can be

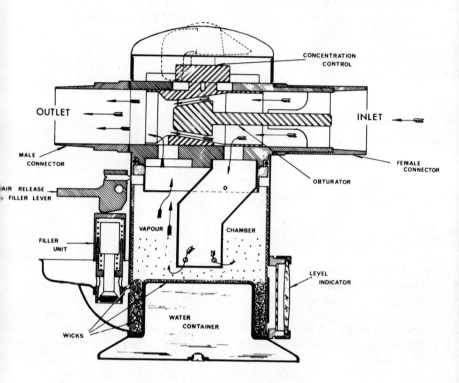

Fig. 4.8   Cross section of the O.M.V.

seen in Figure 4.9. An air by-pass prevents too high a concentration of
vapour building up at low gas flows. The brushed nylon wick is removable
and is capable of absorbing 3 ml liquid halothane. On top of the inhaler is
an annular well which holds about 4 ml of liquid (up to the 'step'). The
wick is stood in this well for a few seconds to soak up the halothane
before being replaced in the bottom of the inhaler, where it is secured by
a bayonet action. Special stops ensure that the unit can only be connected
the right way up on the outlet side of the E.M.O. The resistance to flow is
2–3 mm water at 40 litres per minute.

There are no controls. The unit is operative as soon as the wick has been
replaced and 'turned off' when all the halothane has been used up. Under
hot conditions it may be found that the rate of evaporation of halothane is

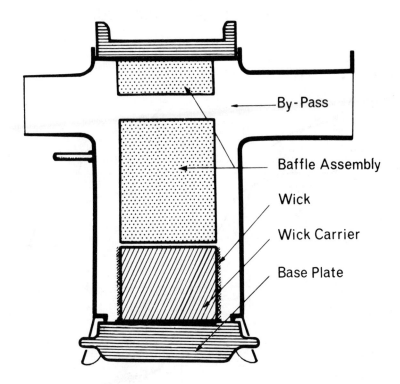

By-Pass

Baffle Assembly

Wick

Wick Carrier

Base Plate

Fig. 4.9   Cross section of the Bryce-Smith Induction Unit (B.S.I.U.)

too great and better results may be obtained by covering half the surface
of the wick with nylon film (cut from a section of lay-flat tubing). This
will not prevent the wick absorbing halothane, but it will reduce the area
available for vaporisation. Good results have also been obtained using
trichloroethylene and chloroform instead of halothane.

Figure 4.10 shows how the concentration of halothane delivered by the
B.S.I.U. varies with time. It delivers between 2 per cent and 4 per cent
halothane for 3–4 minutes. The concentration varies inversely with the
minute volume, so that with a large patient the air flow is so great that only
a low concentration is achieved, while for a small patient the reverse is
true.

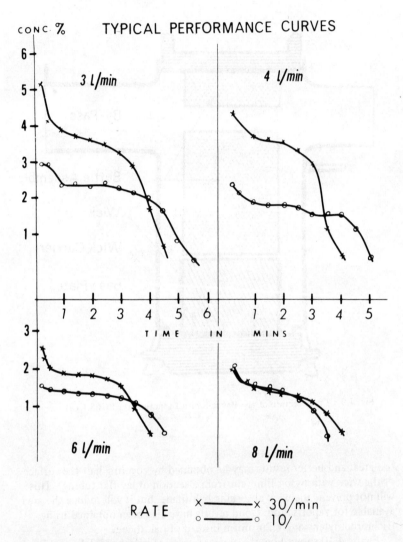

Fig. 4.10 Graphs showing the outputs of halothane from the B.S.I.U. at different minute volumes

Accessories for use with the vaporisers

Bellows units and self-inflating bags

The E.M.O. was originally accompanied by the Oxford Inflating Bellows (O.I.B.) which is shown in Figure 4.11 (Macintosh, 1953). A tap for addition of oxygen is situated at the base of the bellows. This is intended for use only in resuscitation and should always be kept closed during anaesthesia (see below). It weighs 3.5 kg and is 25 cm long by 23 cm high and 18 cm wide. The O.I.B. is essentially a spring loaded concertina bellows with non-return flap valves to ensure that the direction of gas flow is correct and hence that there is no rebreathing of expired air. It was originally intended for use with a simple spring-loaded expiratory valve. This arrangement works well with spontaneous respiration, but for artificial respiration is less satisfactory (see Chapter 5). For this reason a non-rebreathing or inflating valve is usually preferred. Compression of the bellows during artificial respiration will produce full deflection of the valve flaps

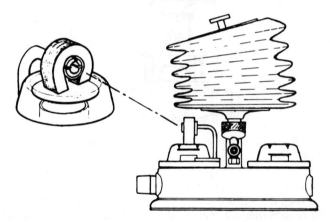

Fig. 4.11   Oxford Inflating Bellows (O.I.B.) The magnet is used to immobilise the distal flap valve when an automatic non-rebreathing valve is used at the patient end

or bobbin during inspiration. In order to draw the bobbin or flaps back and hence to permit the patient to expire to atmosphere, a very small amount of air must pass back up the corrugated tube towards the bellows. If the distal bellows valve is not immobilised, air will be unable to pass back and the non-rebreathing valve will stick in the position of inspiration. The magnet shown in Figure 4.11 is therefore provided for immobilising the distal flap. The magnet *must* be fitted whenever a non-rebreathing valve is used.

Because of these difficulties (see also Chapter 5), a simpler bellows called the Penlon Bellows Unit (P.B.U., Figure 4.12) was developed. This has a single flap valve and was designed specifically for use with a non-rebreathing valve. It must *never* be used with a simple spring loaded expiratory valve (see Chapter 5). It weighs only 1 kg and can be held in the hand or hung from a belt for use in artificial respiration. The latest version has a spring loaded oxygen inlet valve.

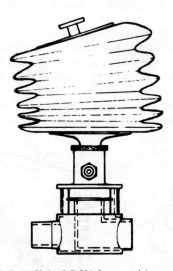

Fig. 4.12   Penlon Bellows Unit (P.B.U.) for use with an automatic non-rebreathing valve.

Both these bellows have internal springs. Press-studs inside the concertinas keep them closed during storage and transport. Both bellows are capable of delivering a volume of about 1300 ml; a 10 cm stroke will deliver about 800 ml. When released, the bellows rise and fall passively with the patient's breathing. These units should be tested for leaks by blocking the outlet and compressing the bellows. The commonest site for a leak is at the base of the concertina, where it is connected to the valve unit with a lock nut and washer.

A special Paediatric Bellows is available for either of these units. It is of smaller diameter and has a full stroke capacity of about 400 ml, making it easier to ventilate small children. It can be fitted by undoing the red plastic lock-nut at the base of the adult bellows. The knurled metal ring is unscrewed and the adult bellows lifted off. The paediatric bellows is substituted, first taking care to ensure that there is a washer inside the central stem, and the knurled ring and lock-nut are tightened.

The E.M.O. is also supplied as an alternative with the Ambu double-ended self-inflating bag. The bag is placed between the vaporisers and the non-rebreathing valve, as shown in Figure 4.13. The bag itself is rather heavy and has to support the weight of two lengths of corrugated tubing, making it rather tiring to use. A much better arrangement is to use the Aga Revivator (Dardel et al., 1966) which employs a light, springy single-ended self-inflating bag in conjunction with the Aga Polyvalve (described

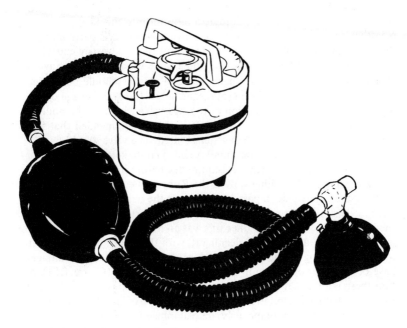

Fig. 4.13   E.M.O. – Ambu Outfit

in the next section). The bag has a volume of 1200 ml and is capable of delivering a tidal volume of up to 1000 ml during an average compression. This unit is the easiest means of giving artificial respiration with the E.M.O. system. It is particularly easy for some trained anaesthetists who paradoxically find it difficult to convert to the use of the bellows, although some people with small hands sometimes prefer to squeeze it between an arm and the body.

Another alternative is to detach the concertina bellows from the O.I.B. and to replace it with a single-ended self-inflating bag on the end of a length of corrugated tubing.

Artificial respiration is fully described in Chapter 5.

Non-rebreathing valves

It is best to use a non-rebreathing valve with the E.M.O. or O.M.V. A non-rebreathing valve, when attached to a facemask or endotracheal tube, will ensure that the patient inspires only from the inhaler and will expire only to the atmosphere. Most valves have the additional virtue of being automatic in operation when used for artificial respiration. An essential feature of any anaesthetic apparatus is that it shall be capable of use for this purpose. With an automatic non-rebreathing valve it is only necessary to compress the bag or bellows in order to blow air into the patient's lungs. No other control is needed which is an obvious advantage, particularly for the non-expert anaesthetist. However, most of these valves are capable of sticking or otherwise malfunctioning and a spare should always be available.

The valves described below, being made of plastics, should be washed out and then sterilised by chemical means only. Heat will damage or destroy them, with the exception of the Aga valve which can be boiled or autoclaved at temperatures up to 135°C. It is recommended that 5 per cent chlorhexidine (Hibitane) in water be used. The valve should be soaked in this solution for five minutes and then shaken out to dry it. Care must be taken to see that it is quite dry before it is used again. The best known non-rebreathing valve is the Ruben. The original version allowed some of the expired air to pass back towards the inhaler, though as this was largely deadspace air (which had not taken part in gas exchange in the lungs), it is doubtful whether this was an important disadvantage. More important is the difficulty of cleaning it, with the risk of dirt accumulating inside and making the bobbin stick (Maggio, 1962). These disadvantages have been largely overcome in the Mark II Ruben valve (Figure 4.14). Note that there is a resuscitation version of this valve which is intended purely for giving artificial respiration. It has no outlet valve and if a patient breathes through it spontaneously, he will inhale only atmospheric air.

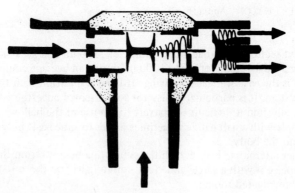

Fig. 4.14   Section of the Ruben Valve, Mark II

Ambu non-rebreathing valves have two silicone rubber flaps in place of a bobbin. They can be dismantled easily by unscrewing the plastic end tapers and lifting off the flaps. The whole can then be washed in soap and water before sterilising. There are two version, the 'E' valve and the low-resistance Hesse valve (Figure 4.15); the latter is the more suitable valve for use with the E.M.O. Attention must be paid to the direction of gas flow because the inlet and outlet tapers are both identical 22 mm cones. It is possible to fit one of the yellow silicone valve elements back-to-front on the expiratory side of the main valve body, instead of on the inlet cone (Kelly, 1968). This will prevent expiration to atmosphere, allowing the patient to rebreathe into the bellows, making him hypoxic (Grogono and Porterfield, 1970). Like the Ruben valve, there is a resuscitation-only version of this valve.

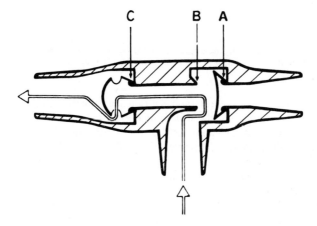

Fig. 4.15   Section of the Ambu valve in the position of expiration. The silicone rubber flap valve at 'A' is closed, while air escapes via hole 'B' and the flap valve at 'C', which is shown open

The Aga Polyvalve Anestor (Figure 4.16) is an automatic non-rebreathing valve, but it is equipped with a length of wide-bore corrugated tubing attached to a single-ended self-inflating bag. When used with the bag the unit is really the Aga Revivator, but with an extra non-return valve on the outlet port. The bag is used solely to provide artificial respiration and may in fact be replaced by an automatic ventilator. It does not alter in size during spontaneous respiration, unlike the bag on a gas machine, nor does it act as a reservoir. The unit is both an anaesthetic non-rebreathing valve and a means of giving artificial respiration, so dispensing with the need for a separate bellows. For resuscitation purposes oxygen can be led into the narrow-bore delivery tube, which lies inside a length of wide-bore

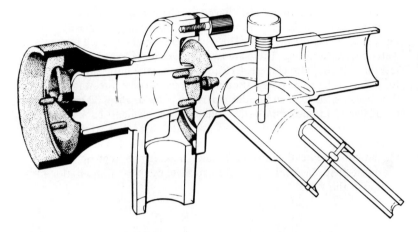

Fig. 4.16   Aga Polyvalve Anestor. The air is taken in from the vaporiser via the tube at the lower right. The upper right tube connects to the self-inflating bag. The patient connection is at the bottom of the picture.

corrugated tubing acting as a reservoir. During anaesthesia the oxygen delivery tube is not used and the wide-bore corrugated tube is attached directly to the outlet of the vaporiser. The Polyvalve is not designed for use with a bellows, but a bellows can be used in place of the bag if the air inlet port of the valve is occluded with a rubber bung to prevent entry of air (which would dilute the anaesthetic mixture).

The Polyvalve Anestor is the simplest and best unit for use with draw-over inhalers and is recommended in preference to the bellows and valve unit described above. The reasons are, firstly, that squeezing of a bag on the end of a length of tubing is the easiest means of giving artificial respiration by hand. Secondly, the valve itself works in a positive manner, with virtually no forward or backward leak, has a low deadspace (3.5 ml), low resistance to flow (less than 3 cm H_2O at 60 litres per minute) and has a low opening pressure without sticking (Johannison, 1966). The disadvantage, both with the Aga and Ambu bags, is that they give no visual indication of respiration.

Many other non-rebreathing valves are made, but for use with a draw-over inhaler it is essential to have one that is suitable for spontaneous as well as artificial respiration. Some types are designed only for inflating the lungs or else only for spontaneous breathing. It is essential to find out exactly how a valve works before using it. It is usually possible to assemble the system incorrectly and the anaesthetist should *always* check the system before use by working the bellows or bag to check the direction of gas flow.

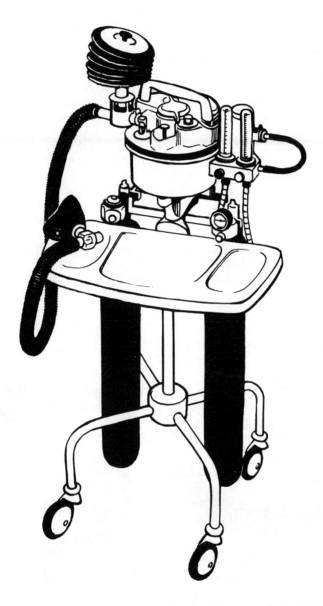

Fig. 4.17   Longworth Hospital Stand. It is shown here with an E.M.O., Mark I two-gas flowmeter unit, P.B.U., Ruben valve and cylinders of nitrous oxide and oxygen with their regulators.

Hospital Stand/Gas Cylinders and Flowmeter Unit

In a hospital or clinic it is convenient to leave the E.M.O. out ready for use. An ordinary small hospital trolley can be used for this purpose. The inhaler with its bellows, facemasks, laryngoscope, bottles of ether, etc. can all be kept in a state of readiness. Alternatively, a special wheeled trolley designed for the E.M.O. is available (Figure 4.17). This has a bracket for the inhaler and a tray for the accessories. Reducing valves for nitrous oxide and oxygen can be mounted on bars at the back. Pin-index yokes for 680 litre (24 cu ft American E size) cylinders are normally provided, but adaptors are available for 1360 litre (48 cu ft) and other cylinders with screw-thread outlets. The manufacturer's instruction book gives details of the assembly procedure.

Flowmeters are needed if gases are to be used. A special two-gas Rotameter unit which allows any proportion of nitrous oxide or oxygen to be added to the inspired mixture is shown in Figure 4.18. This can be of advantage during the induction of anaesthesia (see Chapter 6). If the fresh gas flow is less than the patient's minute volume, air will still be drawn through the inhaler. The Mark I two-gas flowmeter unit shown in Figure 4.17 permits the entry of air through the gravity flap valve and is

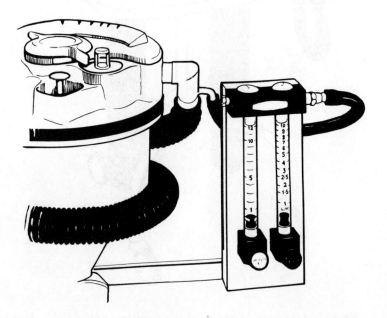

Fig. 4.18   The two-gas flowmeter unit, Mark II. This differs from the Mark I in having a T-piece gas reservoir rather than a gravity-flap inlet valve

plugged directly into the air inlet of the E.M.O. This arrangement can allow the E.M.O. to operate as a plenum (constant gas flow) vaporiser, allowing a lower than indicated concentration of ether to be delivered if the fresh gas flow is less than 10 litres per minute. There is also a danger of the bellows overfilling and a non-rebreathing valve sticking if the fresh gas flow is greater than the patient's minute volume. The Mark II version, which has now superseded the Mark I, fits onto the bar of the hospital stand and delivers the gases to a T-piece with a long corrugated reservoir which is plugged into the air inlet of the vaporiser. The reservoir is filled during expiration with gases which are then consumed by the patient in the next breath.

A special unit designed for use with 'Entonox' (cylinders of pre-mixed

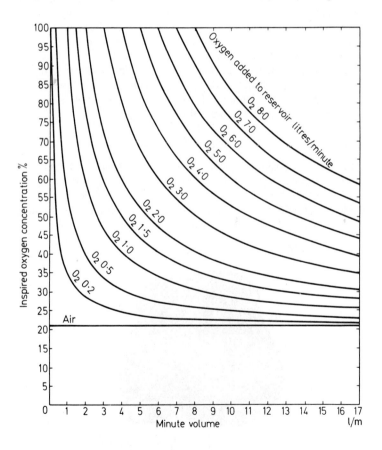

Fig. 4.19   Oxygen enrichment chart

50 per cent nitrous oxide in oxygen) has been developed by Latham and
Parkbrook (1967). It consists of a special regulator (reducing valve) and a
flowmeter with a fine-control valve which will fit the air inlet of an E.M.O.
or O.M.V. It was designed for giving halothane-nitrous oxide-oxygen via a
Magill circuit for dental work. This unit is not compatible with a draw-over
system, but would be a useful flow source when using the E.M.O. or
O.M.V. as constant flow vaporisers in paediatric work, as described in
Chapter 10.

Means of enriching the inspired mixture with oxygen

Oxygen is added to the inhaled air through a narrow delivery tube passed
into the air inlet of the E.M.O. A bubble flowmeter can be used if no other
type is available (Farman, 1961). Care must be taken not to obstruct the
inflow of air into the inhaler either by using too large a tube or with adhesive
tape. However, the best way of introducing oxygen is with the T-piece,
gas reservoir adapter and reservoir tube, which avoids the dilution of
anaesthetic vapour which occurs when oxygen is led directly into the
O.I.B. or P.B.U. The concentration of oxygen achieved will depend
both on the volume added and on the patient's minute volume; the
relationship between these factors is shown in Figure 4.19.

Facemasks

'Everseal' (sizes 1–4) are good under African conditions, (M.I.E.) (Figure
4.20). Connell type masks can be moulded to shape and more nearly
universal in fitting (e.g. B.O.C. 'Contour' Figure 4.21) while the flat
inflatable type is still widely used (Figure 4.22). For infants the Rendell-
Baker masks are easily the best (Figure 10.4, page 149).

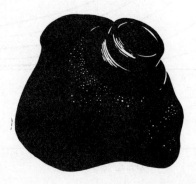

Fig. 4.20   M.I.E. Everseal facemask

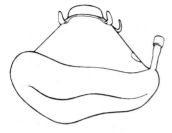

Fig. 4.21   B.O.C. Connell type
anatomical facemask

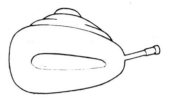

Fig. 4.22   'Flat' type facemask

Dust filter (*H. G. East & Co.*)

Dust and insects can enter the patient's lungs if some form of filter is not
used. It is shown in Figure 4.23 attached via a T-piece oxygen reservoir
to the air inlet of the E.M.O. It may also be attached to the oxygen reservoir
of the flowmeter unit.

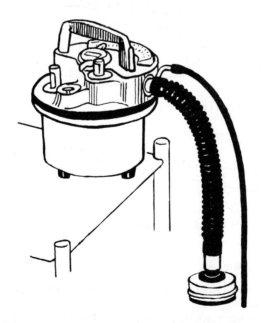

Fig. 4.23   Oxygen T-piece reservoir plugged into the air inlet of the E.M.O.
A dust filter is attached to the end of the reservoir tube

Suction apparatus

This may be foot operated (e.g. Cape or Ambu, Figure 4.24) or electrically operated. An electric sucker with emergency foot operation is available (Cape). Pharyngeal suckers of metal (Yankauer's wide-bore) or sterilisable plastic (e.g. Argyle 1100, Figure 4.25) and whistle tipped catheters complete the set.

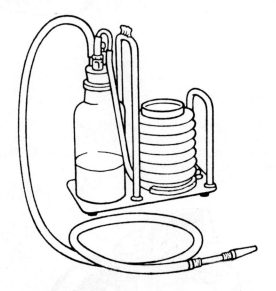

Fig. 4.24   Ambu foot-operated suction pump

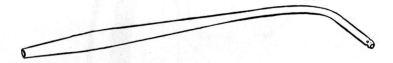

Fig. 4.25   Argyle 1100 pharyngeal suction end

Sponge holding forceps

Although less useful than a sucker, these can be used to mop secretions from the patient's mouth.

A warning is necessary that apparatus made by different manufacturers may not be interchangeable. It is best, therefore, to specify B.S. fittings, made to British Standard 3849 (1965). These are interchangeable with the

U.S. Standard ASA.Z.79. The British Standard specifies a series of 22 mm male outlet cones (usually pointing downstream towards the patient) fitting a series of female cones.

For small children the paediatric cone is of 15 mm diameter, but the order is reversed (i.e. male cones point upstream).

Apparatus used for endotracheal intubation is described in Chapter 5, while paediatric apparatus is covered in Chapter 10 (Anaesthesia in Children).

Chapter Five

Ventilation of the Lungs

Anybody who is going to give an anaesthetic must possess certain skills, the most important of which is the ability to maintain a clear airway. This is an essential part of the care of any unconscious patient, including the anaesthetised patient. The ability to pass an endotracheal tube and to give artificial respiration are also essential if the full benefit of anaesthesia is to be obtained. These techniques will also prove invaluable in resuscitation.

Maintaining a clear airway

Perhaps the most important thing in the whole of anaesthesia is the maintenance of a clear airway. In the unconscious patient this mainly concerns means of preventing the tongue falling back and obstructing the pharynx. This can be achieved in several ways.

Firstly, methods are available to the doctor or nurse which do not depend on instruments. When the patient is supine, the first movement to be performed is extension of the head. This means extending the atlanto-occipital joint and can be achieved by simply grasping the head with one hand and tilting it so that the nostrils point upwards. This has the effect of raising the mandible away from the cervical spine and hence, in spite of the fact that the mouth may remain open, lifting the tongue off the posterior pharyngeal wall. This is illustrated in Figure 5.1. It should be remembered that the tongue is attached via the hyoid bone to the mandible and that anything which raises the mandible away from the posterior pharyngeal wall will lift the tongue at the same time. Very often this manoeuvre alone is successful in clearing an obstructed airway. A small pillow or rolled sheet placed under the neck will help to maintain this position.

However, in some cases this will not be enough and it will be necessary to further raise the mandible by pulling upwards under the point of the jaw, as shown in Figure 5.2. In young adults with a full set of teeth this usually ensures a clear airway. In some adult subjects, and also particularly in young children, it may be necessary to lift the angle of the jaw on either side in order to clear the air passages, as shown in Figure 5.3. To do this it is most convenient to sit at the head of the patient, the position normally

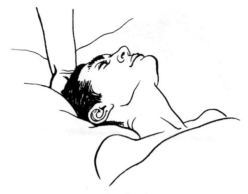

Fig. 5.1   Head-tilt method of clearing the air passages

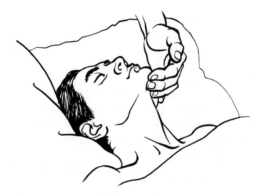

Fig. 5.2   Lifting the point of the jaw to assist clearing the air passages

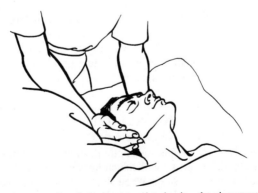

Fig. 5.3   Lifting the angles of the jaw to assist clearing the air passages

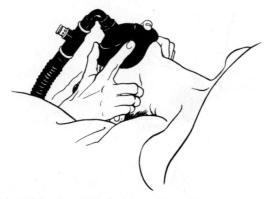

Fig. 5.4   Lifting the angles of the jaw while holding a facemask. Note that
in this case a spring-loaded expiratory valve is being used.

adopted by the anaesthetist, with one's elbows resting on the end of the
operating table. It is then quite easy to lift the angle of the jaw with the
second finger of each hand. It is less tiring to bend the fingers up into a
wedge; the first finger and thumb of each hand will then remain free to
hold on the facemask as shown in Figure 5.4. In edentulous subjects the
jaw closes more than in normal people and these manoeuvres alone may
not ensure a clear airway. The lips prevent air entering, while the tongue
occupies most of the mouth. Although the patient may be able to breathe
in through his nose, the soft palate drops back, forming a one-way valve
and this may prevent him expiring.

If the methods described above prove insufficient, then an oral airway
must be inserted. The best type of airway is the Guedel pattern (B.O.C. or
Portex, Figure 5.5). It should be lubricated before use by applying a little
lubricant to the outer curve. This is then used to lubricate the patient's
lips. The mouth is allowed to drop open momentarily and the airway inserted
with the tip pointing upwards towards the hard palate (see Figure 5.6). It
is then rotated through 180° so that its curve follows that of the soft
palate and the back of the tongue. The airway then comes to lie with its
tip between the base of the tongue and the posterior pharyngeal wall. The
jaw must then be supported as described above. In most patients this will
ensure that the air passages remain clear. The size of the airway will depend
on the size of the patient. Normally a child will require a No. 1, a woman
a No. 2, and a man a No. 3 Guedel, but different manufacturers have
different ways of numbering their airways.

Occasionally in an unconscious patient, or as a result of mismanagement
during anaesthesia, a patient will clench his jaws tightly shut, preventing
the insertion of an oral airway. When this happens it may be necessary to
use a boxwood wedge to force the teeth apart. A mouth gag may then be

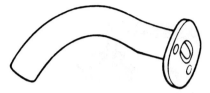

Fig. 5.5   Oral airway, Guedel pattern

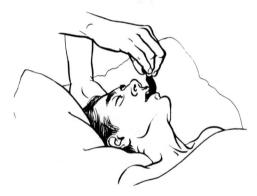

Fig. 5.6   Inserting an oral airway. It is first pointed towards the roof of the mouth and then turned as it is advanced

introduced and used to open the mouth so that an airway can be introduced, or in order to suck blood or vomit from the pharynx. Ferguson's gag, with Acland jaws (Figure 5.7), is the type recommended. It should seldom be needed, but must always be present.

When giving an anesthetic there is the additional problem of obtaining an airtight fit with the facemask while the air passages are kept clear. This requires that the facemask must be pressed on to the face at the same time as the jaw is supported. However, with a little practice this can often be

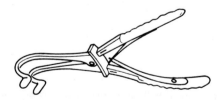

Fig. 5.7   Ferguson's gag, with Acland jaws to assist insertion between the teeth

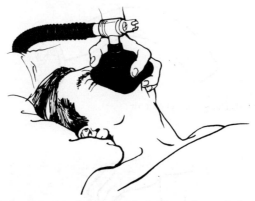

Fig. 5.8 Lifting the point of the jaw while holding a facemask. In this case an Ambu valve is shown

achieved with one hand alone, as shown in Figure 5.8. When this is insufficient, the two-handed method described will usually prove successful.

Various rubber harnesses are available. These hold the facemask on to the patient's face and do not assist the lifting of the jaw. The harness should be placed beneath the patient's head before the anaesthetic is started. It should only be connected up when it is quite certain that the patient is breathing smoothly and that there is no respiratory obstruction (i.e. after reaching surgical anaesthesia). Care should be taken to ensure that the side pieces of the harness arc of equal length and that equal tension is applied when connecting them. In the case of the three cornered Clausen harness (Figure 5.9), the single long arm should be placed so that it passes over the top of the patient's head, while the two shorter side arms pass on either side of the head. With this type of harness a three-hooked ring is necessary. The Connell type of harness has four adjustable straps which fit onto hooks on either side of the facemask (Figure 5.10). A harness should never be used with patients in whom there is the slightest risk of vomiting or regurgitation; they should be intubated whenever possible. This includes the majority of obstetric cases, patients with intestinal obstruction, with bleeding into the mouth or pharynx and patients who have had recent meals. In all these cases it may be necessary to remove the facemask without delay in order to suck out the mouth and a harness would prevent this.

Endotracheal Intubation

Although in many patients it will be simplest and easiest to maintain a clear airway in the manner already described, for a certain proportion of cases endotracheal intubation is required.

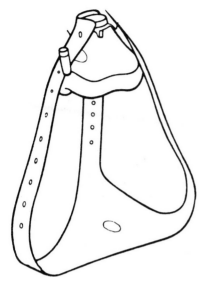
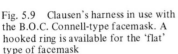

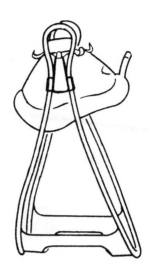

Fig. 5.9   Clausen's harness in use with
the B.O.C. Connell-type facemask. A
hooked ring is available for the 'flat'
type of facemask

Fig. 5.10   Connell's harness which fits
the side hooks of the mask. This type
cannot easily be used with the 'flat'
type of facemask

Indications for endotracheal intubation

1) When a clear airway cannot otherwise be maintained, e.g. due to
anatomical deformities or when depending on an unskilled assistant.

2) In most abdominal operations to protect the lungs from regurgitated
stomach contents. This applies particularly to patients who are vomiting
or who have full stomachs.

3) When artificial respiration is needed (see Chapter 9).

4) For operations in unusual positions, e.g. when the patient has to lie
face-down.

5) For operations in which there is a danger of blood and mucus being
aspirated, such as dental or nasal operations.

6) For operations during which the anaesthetic apparatus must be kept
away from the surgical field, e.g. intra-cranial and ophthalmic procedures,
thyroidectomy.

7) In certain non-surgical conditions. Examples are oedema of the glottis,
prolonged respiratory failure needing artificial respiration, cases requiring
extensive bronchial toilet and in cases of prolonged unconsciousness.

Apparatus for endotracheal intubation

Laryngoscopes

The 130 mm Macintosh adult blade is the most versatile as it can be used on children down to the age of about five (Figure 5.16, page 78). For the smaller children the 105 mm Seward baby blade (Figure 10.6, page 151) is best. For out of the way places a large handle is best as it takes the universally available U2 (American size D) cells. The standard handle, which is the one most commonly seen, takes U11 cells (American size C), while there are smaller handles designed to improve the balance of infant blades. All present-day high-quality blades are autoclavable. A cheaper alternative is an all-plastic laryngoscope with a fixed Macintosh blade (Figure 5.11). This can only be sterilised by boiling or by chemical means provided the batteries are removed first. A paediatric version is also available.

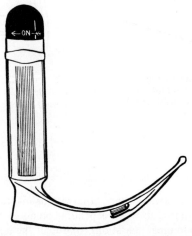

Fig. 5.11   Penlon plastic laryngoscope. The shape of the blade is very similar to the steel Macintosh type

Endotracheal tubes

Sizes 6–10 mm Magill cuffed are used for most purposes. If endotracheal intubation is only performed occasionally, the 'half millimetre' sizes need not be stocked. They are delivered long and have to be cut to size, but beware of making them too short. Table 5.1 gives the average lengths required.

Oxford non-kinking tubes with a built-in right angle bend (Figure 5.12) are best for children and for operations about the head and neck during which an ordinary Magill tube is liable to kink. Sizes 3.5 to 5.5 mm

Table 5.1. Recommended lengths for Endotracheal tubes:

Size of tube in mm	Length in cm	
B.S.	Oral	Nasal
3.0	12	13
3.5	12	13
4.0	13	14
4.5	14	15
5.0	15	16
5.5	16	17
6.0	17	19
6.5	18	21
7.0	19	23
7.5	20	25
8.0	21	27
8.5	23	29
9.0	24	31
9.5	25	–
10.0	26	–
11.0	27	–

This is a guide to the length of endotracheal tubes. The optimal lengths for individual patients will obviously vary.

uncuffed and a full range of cuffed sizes are recommended. They are the correct length and do not need shortening. A malleable introducer is needed to assist the passage of the Oxford type. A range of nasal tubes is useful for patients who cannot be intubated via the mouth. Nasal tubes are uncuffed and have sharper bevels than oral tubes. They have to be cut to size (see Table 5.1). For long-term care a few pre-sterilised plastic cuffed tubes should be kept. A set of cleaning brushes is needed.

Endotracheal connectors

These fit into the endotracheal tubes. Cobb's suction unions, sizes 2, 3 and 4 with rubber bungs (B.O.C.), are best for the adult size tubes. When using an Oxford tube the bung is removed so that the introducer can pass

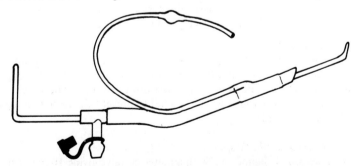

Fig. 5.12   Oxford tube with Cobb connector and introducing stilette

through the connector (Figure 5.12). For children the Rees-modified
Ayre's T-piece is available with special plug-in connectors (Penlon).
Children's equipment is described in Chapter 10.

Catheter mount connector
This joins the endotracheal connector to the non-rebreathing valve. These
items are shown in Figure 5.13.

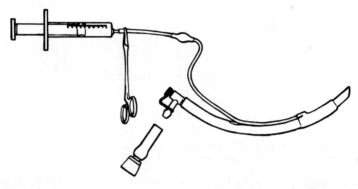

Fig. 5.13   Magill tube with Cobb connector, catheter mount and cuff
inflating syringe

Small artery forceps
Used to pinch the cuff tubing.

10 ml nylon syringe
This should if possible have a combined (Record/Luer) taper which will fit
all types of cuff tubing. Alternatively, special cuff inflators with non-return
valves can be obtained, e.g. the 'Mitchell' (Penlon).

Magill's forceps
These are specially designed to assist the passage of endotracheal or
oesophageal tubes under direct laryngoscopic vision (Figure 5.14).

Lubricant
Ordinary lubricating jelly is essential for endotracheal or oesophageal tubes,
for the introducers for Oxford tubes and sometimes for the laryngoscope.
When a short-acting relaxant is used to assist intubation, it is better to
use local anaesthetic paste (e.g. Lignocaine) to prevent the patient coughing
on the tube afterwards.

Local anaesthetic sprays
Use of an aerosol of lignocaine, with a metering valve giving 10 mg of the
drug for each puff, is a very economical and easy way of spraying the

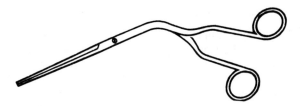

Fig. 5.14   Magill's introducing forceps. These have a double angle to assist their use during laryngoscopy

larynx before intubation. Alternatively, a 5 ml plastic syringe and a stiff 1mm bore venous catheter 10–15 cm long can be used for spraying 2 per cent solution. The special sprays used for this purpose are often more trouble than they are worth. These are shown in Figure 5.15.

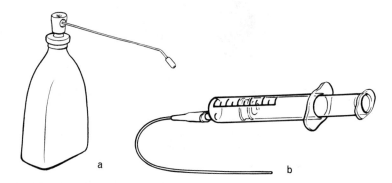

Fig. 5.15a   Aerosol of lignocaine with metering valve, giving 10 mg per puff
Fig. 5.15b   5 ml syringe with fine plastic catheter for spraying the cords with 2 per cent lignocaine

Condenser humidifier

(Mapleson, Morgan and Hillard, 1963.) This consists of a series of layers of stainless steel gauze in a double-sided plastic holder with inlet and outlet tapers to B.S. 3849. It is placed between the endotracheal catheter mount connector and the non-rebreathing valve. As the patient expires about 80 per cent of the moisture condenses on the gauze, but during inspiration it re-evaporates. It thus warms and moistens the inspired air. It also protects the non-rebreathing valve against condensation, which may make it stick (Knight, 1968) and acts as a filter and sputum trap (Collis, 1967). It is easily cleaned, the gauze element being removable for sterilisation. It is shown in use in Figure 5.20, page 81.

Direct vision orotracheal intubation

Before passing the tube either anaesthesia must be well established, to the
level of surgical anaesthesia with adequate relaxation, or relaxation of the
jaw must be provided by a muscle relaxant. In the latter case the lungs
must be well filled with oxygen beforehand (see Chapter 7). It is also
possible to pass a tube under local anaesthesia in patients in whom there
is a contra-indication to intubating under general anaesthesia, such as
laryngeal oedema or anatomical difficulties (see below).

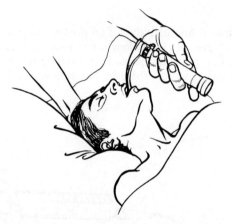

Fig. 5.16   Laryngoscopy – Inserting the Macintosh laryngoscope while the
anaesthetist's right hand extends the patient's head

The curved Macintosh laryngoscope is used in a majority of patients. It
is suitable for adults and children over the age of about five. In patients with
dry mouths it may be necessary to lubricate the end of the blade with
lubricating jelly. The patient's head should be supported on one or two
pillows so that the neck is flexed. With the anaesthetist standing behind the
patient, the head is tilted into the position described in the first section
(shown in Figure 5.1, page 69), using the right hand while the laryngoscope
is held in the left hand (Figure 5.16). The blade should be gently introduced
into the mouth slightly to the right of the midline so as to deflect the
tongue to the left. It is passed down the back of the tongue until the
epiglottis is seen. The laryngoscope is then tilted slightly upwards so that
its tip goes between the epiglottis and the base of the tongue. The tongue
is then lifted out of the line of vision and the larynx should come into
view. The angle between the mouth and the pharynx is thus converted
into a straight line.

Care must be taken not to damage the fauces or the posterior pharyngeal

wall with the tip of the laryngoscope blade. The teeth should also be
treated gently and should not be used as a fulcrum. Difficulties may occur
with patients who have some teeth missing, while loose teeth may easily be
dislodged during intubation.

The appearance of the glottis at laryngoscopy is shown in Figure 5.17.
If the cords are found to be in spasm, either the relaxant has not yet
worked or the patient is not sufficiently deep. In the latter case the
laryngoscope should be removed and the anaesthetic continued until a
sufficient depth of anaesthesia has been reached. Under no circumstances

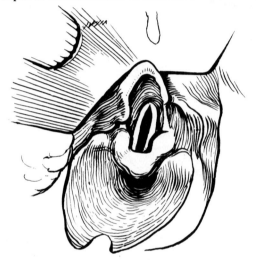

Fig. 5.17   Anaesthetist's view of the larynx. It is not always possible to see
the anterior (upper in this view) ends of the vocal cords. The arytenoid
processes are valuable landmarks during endotracheal intubation. From
a photograph taken with an Olympus fibreroptic endoscopic camera

should the tube be forced through the cords. It may help at this stage to
have an assistant push the larynx backwards to bring it into view. If the
laryngoscope light fails, the larynx can be transilluminated by shining
an electric light through the overlying skin (Tate, 1955).

The larynx and trachea may be sprayed with lignocaine before passing
the tube (Figure 5.18). A dose of 1 mg/kg (five to ten puffs of the aerosol
or 2.5 to 5 ml of 2 per cent lignocaine solution) is usually sufficient. This
will virtually eliminate the possibility of the patient coughing on the tube
or holding his breath after intubation and will help to ensure a smooth
resumption of spontaneous respiration after using a short-acting muscle
relaxant. Local anaesthetic solutions increase the risk of inhaling vomit,
mucus, blood, tooth fragments or other such material during the recovery
period and should therefore be avoided for operations about the mouth

and nose. When the relaxed cords can be seen, the lubricated tube is then passed through the right hand side of the mouth into the trachea under direct vision (Figure 5.19).

The commonest mistake is to pass the tube into the oesophagus. Always check that it has passed in front of the arytenoid cartilages. If it is seen to lie in front of them, it must be in the trachea. An additional check that the tube is in the trachea may be made by listening to the end of the connector. Air will be heard passing in and out of the tube and the warm expired air felt against the skin. In paralysed patients it is necessary to

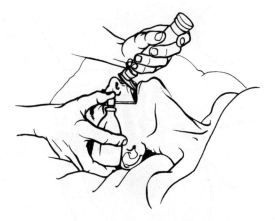

Fig. 5.18   Use of the lignocaine aerosol to spray the larynx before intubation

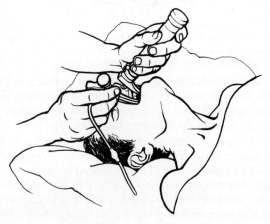

Fig. 5.19   Passing the endotracheal tube. Sometimes this is easier if an assistant presses the larynx backwards

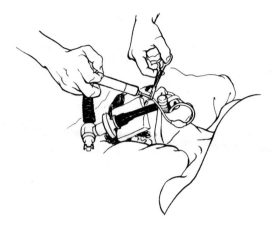

Fig. 5.20　Inflating the cuff while blowing air into the lungs. Just enough air is used to prevent leak-back past the cuff. The patient is protected by a plastic foam pad from pressure from the catheter mount, to which a vapour condenser has been connected

press on the chest in order to expel some air through the endotracheal tube. When the tube is in position, the laryngoscope is removed and an oral airway inserted. The metal-reinforced portion of the airway will act as a mouth prop, preventing the patient biting through the endotracheal tube and obstructing his own airway.

A cuffed tube should be used whenever there is any bleeding into the mouth, when the patient is likely to vomit or regurgitate stomach contents, and when artificial respiration is to be given. To inflate the cuff, a 10 ml syringe is attached to the end of the cuff tubing and air blown into the patient's lungs with the bellows or bag. While pressure is being applied to the lungs in this way, air will be heard bubbling out between the endotracheal tube and the tracheal wall. Air is blown into the cuff with the syringe until the bubbling can no longer be heard or felt. A clip is then applied to the cuff tubing to prevent the air coming out, as shown in Figure 5.20. Some endotracheal tubes are fitted with non-return valves which make a clip necessary. For operations about the nose, mouth or throat, a pharyngeal pack is recommended in addition to soak up the blood. This consists of a length of 5 cm (2 in) saline-soaked ribbon gauze (not bandage, which has loose threads). The laryngoscope is re-inserted into the mouth and the gauze led into the pharynx and packed lightly around the endotracheal tube, using Magill's intubation forceps.

The tube should be firmly fixed in place, as shown in Figure 5.20. A length of 5 cm (2 in) bandage may be passed behind the patient's neck, one turn taken round the suction arm of the endotracheal connector, and then tied. Alternatively, a length of adhesive tape may be applied to hold the endotracheal connector on to the face. It is usually necessary to attach the catheter mount connector before doing this. In either case, a pad of foam plastic or a few gauze mops should be placed between the connector and the patient's face to prevent pressure on the skin. Once the tube has been passed, it should lie snugly and comfortably.

It is preferable to employ a vapour condenser between the catheter mount and the non-rebreathing valve (see above). This is of particular importance in dry climates where there is a definite danger that the tracheal mucosa will dry out and tracheal and bronchial secretions become dry and viscid when an endotracheal tube is used.

Difficulties in intubation

Difficulty may be experienced in patients whose anatomical shape is unfavourable. These include those with short muscular necks, receding lower jaws, protruding upper incisors or long high-arched palates. Certain pathological conditions also present difficulties. Trismus may be due to arthritis of the temporo-mandibular joints, cancrum oris (especially in the late stage when scarring predominates) or to cellulitis of the sub-maxillary region. Difficulty in extending the head and neck may accompany spondylitis of the cervical spine or scarring of the infra-mandibular skin following burns, making it difficult to get a view of the larynx. Lastly, tumours of the mandible or of the maxilla may interfere with the passage of a laryngoscope. In these patients careful pre-operative assessment is necessary to decide whether or not the patient will be able to breathe adequately when anaesthetised with a facemask. When this seems possible, it may be preferable to take the patient down with ether to the stage of surgical anaesthesia before attempting intubation. This is because difficulties may arise in inflating the lungs after the use of a relaxant if intubation is unsuccessful. It is usually helpful in difficult cases to employ a stilette to guide the endotracheal tube. This can be used with either the Magill or the Oxford type of tube. It is lubricated well and then passed down the tube via a suction connector. The stilette is malleable and the tube can therefore be shaped easily. The tip is allowed to stick out at 2 cm beyond the end of the tube. The laryngoscope is then introduced into the mouth as well as possible, while an assistant presses the larynx back. The tube is advanced carefully until the tip of the stilette has passed between the cords. It will be found that the rest of the tube will follow without much difficulty. The assistant can feel the tube passing down the trachea because its tip rubs against the cartilagenous rings, making it vibrate. The position of the tube is then checked in the manner described above.

Intubation under local anaesthesia

When it seems unlikely that the anaesthetised patient will be able to breathe
through a facemask without respiration becoming obstructed, intubation
should be attempted under local analgesia. The patient is asked to suck
a local anaesthetic lozenge half an hour before the procedure begins. The
lips and tongue are then sprayed with 2 per cent lignocaine or with a
lignocaine aerosol, and after a couple of minutes the laryngoscope is gently
introduced into the mouth. The remainder of the tongue and the posterior
surface of the epiglottis are sprayed. The base of the tongue is then elevated
until the larynx can be visualised and the larynx and trachea sprayed
with local analgesic. The laryngoscope is then withdrawn until any coughing
has ceased. Alternatively 5 ml of 1 per cent lignocaine may be injected into
the trachea via a needle passed through the crico-thyroid membrane.
The laryngoscope is reintroduced after a couple of minutes and the tube
passed. This procedure may be very uncomfortable for the patient in spite
of the local analgesia. Sedation with diazepam 10 mg by intramuscular
injection or about 5 mg intravenously may be effective while droperidol
5 mg intravenously may help to prevent movement. An assistant should be
standing by to hold the patient's arms so as to prevent him clutching at the
laryngoscope or at the anaesthetist's hands. Constant encouragement should
be given to the patient during the procedure.

Nasal intubation

An alternative method for patients with trismus or tumours of the mandible
is to pass the endotracheal tube through the nose. This technique is also
useful for operations about the mouth and throat, or when an oral tube will
be in the surgeon's way. Usually the tube required will be one size smaller
than would be the case for oral intubation. It is possible to pass a cuffed
tube through the nose if a sufficiently small size is employed. The tube
should be very well lubricated beforehand. A nasal tube will require to be
somewhat longer than the usual oral tube as will be seen in Table 5.1, and
it is usual to select one that has recently arrived from the manufacturer and
has not been cut too short. The tip of the nasal tube is also more sharply
pointed (with a 30° bevel) than an oral tube. Nasal intubation may be
difficult or impossible in patients with nasal blockage. It is wise to instil
vaso-constrictor nose drops before passing the tube, so as to shrink the
mucosa.

    Anaesthesia should be induced and the patient either taken to the stage
of surgical anaesthesia with ether or else permitted to breathe oxygen for
two minutes before being given a short-acting muscle relaxant as described
in Chapter 7. The patient's head is placed on one or two pillows, the head
tilted and the neck and upper chest are bared. It is best to control the
movement of the tube with the right hand and to tilt the head of the

patient with the left hand. The tube is introduced into the right nostril and passed directly backwards along the floor of the nasal cavity. It may need to be rotated from time to time to overcome obstruction from the turbinates. Undue force should never be used because bleeding often results. It is advanced steadily until its tip is in the pharynx. At this point the breath sounds will be heard through the tube, particularly if the other nostril is occluded. The commonest fault, as in all intubation, is to let the tube pass into the oesophagus. If this happens during blind nasal intubation it suggests that the head is too much flexed on the neck. If the tip of the tube passes into the pyriform fossa, it will raise the overlying skin lateral to the thyroid cartilage. The tube should then be withdrawn a little and rotated in the appropriate direction. It is essential during nasal intubation that the neck of the patient should be exposed so that the position of the tip of the tube can be detected by watching the skin. When the tube is passed through the glottis, it will often be felt to snap past the cords. It will also be seen to distort the anterior wall of the trachea as it passes.

When passing a nasal tube for routine oral operations it is usually possible to use the laryngoscope in the ordinary way. The tube can then be manoeuvred through the glottis by manipulating its proximal end or by using Magill's intubation forceps. A throat pack is required (see above) if there is any risk of aspiration of mucus or blood into the trachea.

Complications of endotracheal intubation

1) Kinking of the tube. This is likely to happen with an old and worn out Magill tube, when the tube is too long and is left hanging out of the patient's mouth, when the head is moved, particularly flexed, or when the tube is not fixed in place properly.

2) Intubation of the right main bronchus. This fault commonly occurs in patients in whom an unshortened tube is passed. After intubation the chest should be auscultated to ensure that air entry is equal on both sides. If it remains undetected the patient will become cyanosed because the unventilated lung will continue to be perfused with blood. Carbon dioxide will be retained and the work of breathing will become greater. This will exhaust the spontaneously breathing patient.

3) Blockage of the tip of the tube. This is caused by apposition of the bevel to the tracheal wall. It is most likely to happen in a patient whose trachea is deviated, for example by an enlarged thyroid.

4) Obstruction due to the cuff. If the cuff is over-inflated, it may either compress the tube or herniate down beyond the tip, blocking the opening. Before attempting to withdraw the tube, the cuff should be deflated and the respiration again checked.

5) Disconnection of the endotracheal catheter mount connector. This will occur if worn catheter mount tubing is used.

6) Damage: Dislodged teeth, lacerations of the lips, fauces or pharyngeal wall, damage to the cords or cricoid ring (in children) and ulceration of the lips, tongue, cricoid ring or tracheal mucosa during prolonged intubation may all occur.

7) Postoperative complications. It is common for patients to have a slight soreness of the throat accompanied by a husky voice, for a few hours after operation. This usually disappears by the next day. Occasionally, presumably as a result of traumatic intubation, granulomatous polyps grow on the vocal cords.

Artificial respiration

This is sometimes known as intermittent positive pressure respiration or controlled ventilation.

By virtue of its bellows, the E.M.O. apparatus can be used for artificial respiration in any situation. This applies equally to the O.I.B. (Oxford Inflating Bellows) and the Penlon Bellows Unit (P.B.U.). In either case, an automatic non-rebreathing valve is essential. Alternatively, a self-inflating bag may be used. The Aga Polyvalve Anestor is the best one for this purpose because the bag is on a side tube and is therefore easier to handle. This apparatus is described in Chapter 4. The indications for artificial respiration during anaesthesia with relaxants are discussed in Chapter 8.

Artificial respiration consists of two distinct phases. First, air is blown into the patient's lungs (inspiration). Secondly, the air is allowed to escape from the lungs (expiration). While this may seem obvious, in practice it is often difficult to remember to allow sufficient time for expiration. The movement of the chest should always be watched and it must be seen to expand during inspiration. During expiration, make absolutely sure that the next breath does not begin until the chest has emptied. Failure to allow sufficient time for expiration will lead to a high mean intra-thoracic pressure, which will have an adverse effect on the circulation. Mushin et al. (1969) recommended that the duration of expiration should be at least twice that of inspiration.

When using a non-rebreathing valve it should be remembered that the valve is effectively operated by the movements of the bellows or bag. With most types of automatic non-rebreathing valve, it is possible by gentle pressure to blow air across the valve and out through the expiratory port instead of into the patient's lungs. In the case of the Ruben valve, which has a hard plastic bobbin, the bobbin can be made to vibrate rapidly to and fro, making a juddering noise. In either of these cases ventilation won't be effective. The inspiratory movement should therefore begin smartly and continue throughout inspiration as a firm and definite compression of the bag or bellows. Similarly, at the beginning of expiration, it is possible to lift the bellows so slowly that the valve remains in the inspiratory position and air is allowed to pass back up the tubing towards the vaporiser, instead of out to the atmosphere. For this reason inspiration should end, not with the bellows held down, but with a sudden upward movement which is continued until the bellows has been refilled with air for the next breath. Similarly, the bag should be allowed to re-expand immediately. A pause for expiration must then be allowed.

Movement of the bellows during artificial respiration can be characterised by the triple movements, DOWN-UP-PAUSE. This rhythm is essential if effective artificial ventilation is to be given. Figure 5.21 emphasises these movements. Paradoxically, it is probably more difficult for experienced anaesthetists (who are used to squeezing the bags on gas machines) than for non-experts. The technique is different from that used with a gas machine and anaesthetic bag. The feel of the bellows is very direct and many will prefer the Aga unit for this reason.

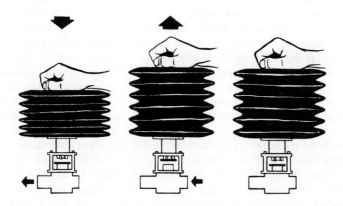

Fig. 5.21   This shows the positions of the anaesthetist's hand and the bellows valve flap during inspiration (DOWN), the start of expiration (UP) and the end of expiration (PAUSE). The P.B.U. is shown for the sake of simplicity

When giving artificial respiration with a facemask, the position of the head should be adjusted as described in the earlier section on the care of the airway. At the same time the facemask must be held in close contact with the patient's face, as shown in Figure 5.22, in order to achieve an airtight seal. With practice this is not difficult. If artificial respiration is attempted in the presence of an obstructed airway, the stomach will be inflated with air. When this happens there is a distinct risk of sudden regurgitation of air and gastric juice, which may then become inhaled. This complication can be prevented by passing an endotracheal tube. If artificial respiration is likely to be prolonged, then an endotracheal tube should always be passed.

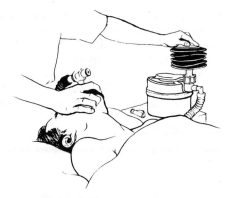

Fig. 5.22   Inflating the lungs with the Penlon bellows, non re-breathing valve and facemask

A word of warning should be given about the use of a spring-loaded expiratory valve with the O.I.B. This bellows unit was designed before automatic non-rebreathing valves were introduced. Clearly, in order to blow air into the lungs, the valve must be screwed down (i.e. shut). Air cannot then escape via the valve so it is necessary to lift the facemask in order to let it out (Macintosh, 1953). A secure fit of the mask must then be obtained before the next breath can be given. When an endotracheal tube is in place, an endotracheal connector with a suction limb, such as the Cobb or Portex type, must be used. The suction hole is occluded with a finger during inspiration. In either case this is a complicated and difficult procedure which is not to be recommended. The magnet on the O.I.B. should *never* be used to immobilise the distal flap valve when a spring loaded expiratory valve is used. Spring loaded valves should *never* be used with the P.B.U. (Penlon Bellows Unit). In either case rebreathing into the bellows would occur. (A few spring loaded valves have a twisting action rather than a screw thread. Some of these have proved faulty, shutting spontaneously during the course of anaesthesia — Das Gupta and Deval, 1970; Sugg, 1970).

It is difficult in the absence of any measuring device to assess the volume of ventilation required by the patient. Under-ventilation with air will lead to development of cyanosis, but a moderate degree of over-ventilation will not be harmful. In fact, because there is an increase in the ratio of physiological deadspace to tidal volume, a large minute volume is needed by the artificially ventilated patient. Very large minute volumes will have an adverse effect on the circulation, by abolishing the thoracic pump mechanism and by interfering with pulmonary capillary blood flow. The lowering of the carbon dioxide tension will decrease cardiac output and cause cerebral vaso-constriction. However, in clinical practice, the dangers of under-ventilation exceed those of over-ventilation.

A spirometer, such as the Wright Respirometer or the Parkinson-Cowan dry gas spirometer, can be fitted to the outlet of the non-rebreathing valve. The Wright Respirometer is more convenient because it is small enough to be fitted directly onto the outlet of the valve. A 10 cm stroke of the adult bellows will deliver about 800 ml, while the Aga bag can deliver up to 1000 ml.

Artificial ventilation in the anaesthetised patient is discussed more fully in Chapter 8.

Ventilators

To obtain the full benefit of the muscle relaxant technique described in Chapter 9, it is best to have an automatic ventilator. The advantages are that a machine is consistent in its work and does not get tired, and that the anaesthetist's hands are free to attend to his drugs, intravenous fluids and so on.

There are many ventilators on the market, few of which are simple or cheap enough to be useful in the sort of conditions considered here (Collis, 1967). It is most convenient to employ electrically-driven machines because electricity is the most widely available power source. Those described here are essentially motorised bellows. The electric motors are of the sparkproof induction type, but the switches are capable of igniting ether vapour and should be removed if ether is to be used. However, trichloroethylene, halothane and methoxyflurane are all non-flammable and provide safe and effective alternatives to ether (see Chapter 8). In no case does the vapour come into contact with the motors. Both the machines described here are very simple and robust and require very little maintenance. Occasional oiling of mechanical parts is needed. The bellows may need to be replaced, but in both cases the bellows units can be removed for cleaning.

East-Radcliffe M2 and B2

In essence this functions as a motorised version of the Penlon Bellows Unit (P.B.U.) and is shown in Figure 5.23. The bellows is lifted by an arm and then allowed to descend, blowing air into the lungs. Weights are placed on top of the bellows, the applied pressure being adjustable by altering the number of weights. The volume of air blown into the lungs (the tidal volume) during each breath is determined by the compliance (volume:pressure relationship) of the lungs and chest wall. If the compliance is reduced (e.g. by an assistant leaning on the patient's chest), the volume delivered by the ventilator will also be reduced. This is because the machine generates a constant pressure during inspiration. It can deliver up to 1200 ml in one breath. A non-rebreathing valve, such as the Ambu, should be used in the normal way in conjunction with a condenser humidifier, as described

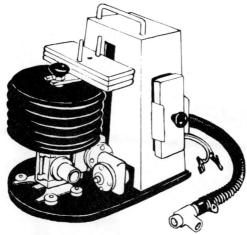

Fig. 5.23   The East-Radcliffe M2 Ventilator

above. The frequency of respiration is fixed at 19 breaths per minute. The duration of inspiration can be adjusted by turning a knob. This is used to prevent the lungs being held inflated after the bellows has descended. If this were to happen, it would have a 'tourniquet' effect, impeding the flow through the pulmonary capillaries.

The bellows can be removed by unscrewing a knob, either for cleaning or in order to perform hand ventilation, in which case it acts in the same way as the P.B.U. There is an oxygen inlet nipple beneath the bellows, intended for use in resuscitation. For use in anaesthesia, the bellows is connected to a vaporiser (E.M.O. or O.M.V.) by a length of corrugated hose. The E.M.O. is placed at a lower level than the ventilator so that any ether vapour which leaks out will not drop onto the electrical parts. It is essential that all connections are leak proof. The exhaust from the non-rebreathing valve should be led to the floor via another length of corrugated hose.

The ventilator is supplied with a choice of motors. The M2 has a mains voltage AC induction motor, and the B2 has a 12 volt DC motor. The latter is designed to work off a car battery for transporting patients by ambulance, etc. Both models weigh 14 kg and cost about £100.

The Cape Minor

This ventilator is also simple to operate. A mains voltage electric motor drives a bellows via an adjustable crank, which varies the tidal volume up to 1300 ml. The frequency is set at 15 breaths per minute. The volume delivered is independent of the compliance of the lungs and chest wall. The Aga Polyvalve is used, the ventilator taking the place of the bag, as shown in Figure 5.24. A condenser humidifier should be used to stop the valve

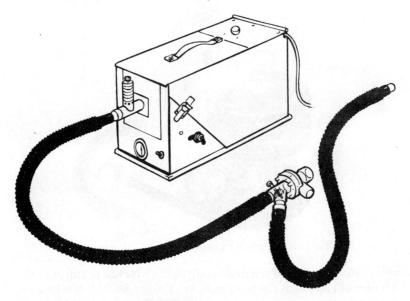

Fig. 5.24   The Cape Minor Ventilator

getting wet. The E.M.O. or O.M.V. is connected to the inspiratory limb of the valve. Again the E.M.O. should be placed below the ventilator to eliminate the risk of ether vapour dropping onto the motor. The bellows can be removed for cleaning. When hand ventilation is required, the corrugated tubing has to be removed from the ventilator and the bag re-attached. There is an oxygen inlet nipple for use in resuscitation and for ward use. The outlet is fitted with an adjustable weighted blow-off valve to limit the applied pressure. A pressure gauge is available as an option. The ventilator weighs 13 kg and costs about £120.

Chapter Six

Pre-operative Preparation

The patient should be welcomed to the hospital and told what to expect concerning the operation to be performed, the arrangements for the day of operation and how he will be given the anaesthetic. It is important to adopt a calm, confident attitude, telling him that he will be given an injection or something to breathe to send him to sleep. He should be warned how long he is likely to remain asleep afterwards, and whether he will wake up with an intravenous drip, a naso-gastric tube or any other such temporary inconvenience. Patients are naturally frightened, both about their operations and about the anaesthetic, particularly having masks on their faces, loss of self control and vomiting. Everything possible should be done to allay these fears and a few words of explanation can save a lot of sedation.

Assessment of the patient's condition

The patient should be carefully questioned and examined before the operation. The history should elicit not only factors pertaining to his surgical condition but should cover his general health as well. In particular, the anaesthetist should ask about his respiratory and circulatory status. Any respiratory disease may seriously interfere with inhalation anaesthesia; particular points to ask about are heavy smoking, chronic cough, production of sputum, asthma and breathlessness. Circulatory disease is equally important and the patient should be asked about ankle oedema, nocturnal or effort dyspnoea, postural faintness, angine pectoris and acute or chronic blood loss. Any other illnesses and previous hospital admissions should be noted, especially the patient's experiences of earlier anaesthetics. He should be asked about any treatment he is now receiving and whether he has reacted adversely to any drugs in the past. Assessment of the patient's condition must always take into account the local pattern of disease.

A general physical examination should be performed. The appearance of the patient should be noted, including his build (normal, obese or emaciated) and mental state (alert, anxious, lethargic, semiconscious or unconscious). The colour of his conjunctival mucosae should be examined for anaemia, cyanosis or jaundice. The mouth should be examined carefully for loose teeth which may be knocked out by a laryngoscope or oral airway (inhalation of a tooth may be followed by the formation of a lung abscess). Tumours of the jaw, tongue or neck may obstruct respiration or interfere with the passage of an endotracheal tube. The patient's state of hydration should be assessed from his mucosae, skin and urine output. A sample of urine should be tested for acidity, specific gravity and for the presence of glucose and albumen. In a hot climate the urinary chloride level should be estimated as a guide to rehydration.

The anaesthetist, in examining the respiratory system, should be interested in the shape and movement of the chest, in signs of sputum retention and lower airways obstruction and in focal signs suggesting areas of collapse or consolidation. It is particularly important not to miss a pneumothorax or pleural effusion. It must also be remembered that large abdominal tumours will interfere seriously with breathing when the patient lies down. If there is doubt about the physical signs, an X-ray picture should be obtained.

Examination of the cardiovascular system aims to reveal conditions in which tissue perfusion is likely to become inadequate during anaesthesia and surgery. The blood pressure should always be taken while the patient is sitting at rest. Postural hypotension will occur in the oligaemic patient. If the blood pressure is taken with the patient supine, this sign, which indicates the need for urgent fluid replacement, will not be elicited. Even if the level is normal, this measurement will be valuable later when assessing the effect of premedicant and anaesthetic drugs. The heart rate and rhythm should be noted. Cardiac enlargement will suggest a considerable degree of organic change, although in endomyocardial fibrosis the heart may not be enlarged even when the ventricles are grossly reduced in size. Signs of cardiac failure may be present. However, the most sensitive criteria of reduced circulatory reserve are effort dyspnoea and postural hypotension. Patients with these symptoms are very likely to become hypotensive under any form of general anaesthetic.

Intercurrent disease

Although the risk associated with a properly conducted anaesthetic is small, it is desirable to treat the conditions discussed above if time is available. In the case of elective operations, treatment should be started when it is first decided to do the operation. Correction of anaemia and treatment of heart failure or of lung infections are examples of this approach. For other patients, operations will not be possible until their conditions have improved. Examples of this are the correction of dehydration, metabolic acidosis or haemorrhage and the treatment of severe chest infections. In an emergency it may be considered essential to proceed to operation knowing that the patient has severe intercurrent disease which has not or cannot be treated. The doctor must then decide whether the risk is justified. Generally speaking, it will be if the operation is life saving.

Patients who are already receiving treatment may be at risk because of their treatment. Drugs used in the treatment of hypertension exert their effect by reducing sympathetic nervous system activity. General anaesthesia will tend to augment this effect and marked falls of blood pressure may be encountered. The blood pressure usually remains within the normal range during ether anaesthesia, but hypotensive drugs will reduce both this effect and the ability of the patient to maintain his blood pressure when the circulating blood volume is reduced. Halothane anaesthesia may be associated with a fall of arterial pressure, even in normal patients. A useful clinical guide is that if a patient experiences postural hypotension while on treatment, he is likely to become hypotensive while under anaesthesia. The dose of hypotensive drug will therefore need to be reduced. Patients receiving alpha-methyl dopa usually present no difficulty, whereas those on the alpha-adrenergic blocking agents such as bethanidine and guanethidine are vulnerable to the hypotensive affect of anaesthesia, as are those taking reserpine. Patients taking beta-adrenergic blocking drugs are also likely to become hypotensive under ether anaesthesia (see Chapter 3). Diuretics present no direct hazard and may be continued, but the thiazide group may cause excessive potassium loss, leading to potassium depletion unless potassium supplements are given.

Diabetics on oral treatment present no difficulty, but those receiving insulin deserve special care. Patients on long-acting insulin should be changed to two daily doses of soluble insulin. Oral intake must be avoided for six hours before the operation. For well established patients on small doses (under 20 units a day), it is best to operate in the early morning, omitting both food and the morning dose of insulin. The evening dose of insulin is only given when it is certain that the patient is able to take food. More severe cases, and those unable to take food, should be given intravenous 5 per cent glucose with 10 units of insulin in every 500 ml bottle, starting at least one hour before operation. Patients with ketosis will require oral or intravenous alkali (sodium bicarbonate) to correct their metabolic acidosis. The use of ether is normally associated with hyperglycaemia. In any event all urine specimens, pre- and post-operative, should be tested for glucose and ketones. For all major procedures an indwelling urinary catheter should be used to obtain samples during operation. If more than 0.2 per cent glucose is present, insulin 5 units should be given intravenously. If there is any doubt about the patient's condition, or if no urine sample is obtainable, the blood sugar level should be estimated with Dextrostix reagent strips.

Patients on psychotropic drugs may present some difficulty. Tranquillisers, particularly those in the phenothiazine group, will cause peripheral vasodilation and a fall in arterial pressure under anaesthesia in some patients, with potentiation of the effect of anaesthetic drugs. On the other hand, if treatment is withdrawn for a period before operation, the patient may become very anxious and require greater than normal doses of anaesthetics. It is better to keep a patient on his normal treatment and to employ the minimum effective doses of anaesthetics, with repeated small doses of analgesics post-operatively. Monoamine oxidase inhibitors slow the rate of breakdown of noradrenaline at nerve endings so that its level remains higher than normal and sympathomimetic drugs, including vasopressors and possibly ether, and sympathetic reflexes such as the hypertensive response to endotracheal intubation, will be potentiated and the patient's arterial pressure may rise to an alarming level. These drugs are not highly specific and also inhibit certain hepatic enzymes with the result that opioids (particularly pethidine) may be potentiated, leading to hypotension and prolonged unconsciousness. When a monoamine oxidase inhibitor is withdrawn, it takes two weeks for newly formed enzyme to reach a normal level in the body. Tricyclic anit-depressants are not known to be dangerous to the anaesthetised patient.

Patients receiving steroid treatment will require extra doses when having operations. For this reason any patient on such treatment or who has recently had a course of steroids is assumed to be steroid dependent and is given extra dosage. Intramuscular or intravenous hydrocortisone may be given beforehand, but acts for little more than the period of the operation, with the risk that hypotension may develop suddenly in the post-operative period. Where possible it is preferable to give double the patient's normal daily dose by mouth about four hours before operation. If hypotension with bradycardia (i.e. not due to oligaemia) develops during or after operation, 100 mg hydrocortisone should be given intravenously. In these cases medication should continue with gradually decreasing dosage in the post-operative period.

Intravenous fluid therapy

This can be considered under three headings. First, the maintenance of a normal physiological balance in the patient undergoing surgery. Secondly, the correction of pathological disturbances of fluid and electrolyte balance. Thirdly, the replacement of blood loss. Fluid and electrolyte balance and the blood volume were discussed in Chapter 2.

Normal fluid balance

The patient about to have an operation should take no food for six hours and no drink for two to four hours. This is to ensure an empty stomach and so to reduce the risk of vomiting. Only a minimum quantity of fluid is allowed to accompany oral premedication. The duration of the operation will often be two hours or more, followed by a variable period, often as long as four hours, during which the patient will feel too sleepy to take much. So for many patients as long as ten hours will pass during which time they will be unable to take oral fluids. Fluids should only be withheld in the immediate pre-operative period. There is no point in denying moderate amounts of water to injured patients on the way to hospital, particularly if a long and difficult journey has to be undertaken (Boulton and Cole, 1968), although these patients may also be suffering from functional extracellular fluid (i.e. electrolyte) loss.

Insensible fluid loss in hospital patients in the tropics is about 1.7 litres per day (Badoe, 1968), representing about one thirtieth of total body water, but will be less than this in a temperate climate. The loss is related to environmental conditions and to the area of the skin and is about one litre per square metre per day, representing for an average adult about 1 ml per kg body weight per hour. An intravenous infusion will compensate for this loss, although of course the patient's requirements will be greater than this because of fluid loss by other routes. There are additional advantages in the use of an infusion. It gives the anaesthetist instant access to the bloodstream for drugs. Transfusion of blood may be needed, possibly urgently, and valuable time will be saved if a drip is already running. For patients having abdominal operations, particularly on the bowel, naso-gastric drainage may be required, necessitating intravenous infusion of fluid. Moreover, the patient is relieved during the post-operative period of his sense of thirst and dryness of the mouth and of the need to take frequent small sips of water. The ability to take an adequate volume of oral fluid is limited for many hours after operation. Lastly, the provision of sufficient fluid intake will ensure an adequate urine output and will protect against renal failure.

The choice of fluid

The main fluid loss during operation consists of extracellular fluid (see Chapter 2) and therefore a balanced electrolyte solution should be given. Lactated Ringer's solution or Hartmann's solution (containing approximately 130 mEq sodium, 5 mEq potassium, 110 mEq chloride and 30 mEq lactate per litre) is best for this purpose. This will prevent any fall in serum sodium level resulting from loss of extracellular fluid and the consequence reduction in renal sodium excretion.

The aim should be to maintain a normal fluid intake during the day of operation and afterwards until the patient can again take fluid by mouth. In the normal adult having an operation it should be infused at the rate of 2 ml per kg per hour, equal to about 3 litres per day. The amount given should be enough to maintain a urine output of not less than 30 ml per hour and preferably 50 ml per hour. When blood and fluid are lost during operation, this additional loss should be replaced at least on a 'drop for drop' basis (Boulton and Cole, 1968a). This applies where blood is not available for transfusion, although it should be remembered that electrolyte solutions will be distributed evenly throughout the extracellular space and will not simply remain in the vascular compartment. Young children and infants may require up to 5 ml per kg per hour because of their relatively large surface (i.e. skin) area.

In the post-operative period, assuming that extracellular fluid and blood volume deficits have been replaced, the need is simply for replacement of insensible water loss and urine output, which together amount to 2000 2500 ml per day in an adult (1.5 ml per kg per hour). This should be given in the form of 2.5 per cent glucose with 0.45 per cent saline. Fluid aspirated from a naso-gastric tube or wound drain should be replaced by an equal volume of 0.9 per cent saline (sodium chloride). In either case the patient should receive 40 mEq potassium (as potassium chloride) per day to replace the urinary potassium loss.

Correction of disturbances of fluid and electrolyte balance

Extracellular fluid losses

These changes are distributional and are therefore primarily volume changes, unaccompanied by changes in ionic concentration. They may consist of measurable external losses which should be replaced with an equal volume of fluid of similar composition. The importance of careful charting of fluid intake and output cannot be overestimated. The composition of various fluids is given in Table 6.1. Ascitic fluid and wound drainage will consist in whole or part of serum transudate which will contain, in addition to the ions given in the table, 20—40 g of protein per litre. Gastro-intestinal fluids have rather higher potassium concentrations than ECF (plasma), while gastric fluid will be richer in hydrogen ions. Problems arise when the

Table 6.1. Composition of body fluids

Fluid	pH	Na^+ mEq/litre	K^+ mEq/litre	Cl^- mEq/litre
Stomach	1.5	20–80	5–20	50–155
Bile	5.7–8.6	120–160	3–15	80–120
Pancreatic juice	7.5–8.0	110–140	3–15	40–80
Duodenum	4.7–6.5	75–140	4–15	70–135
Jejunum	6.2–7.3	105–145	6–29	90–135
Ileum	–	110–140	4.5–14	95–120
Plasma	7.4	130–150	3.5–5.5	90–105
Serum transudate urine	7.4	144	4.9	112

loss is not measurable. In this case reliance must be placed on the clinical signs mentioned in Chapter 2, remembering that the commonest fault is to underestimate the loss. Fluid should be infused at the rate of one to two litres per hour until the signs return to normal and urine output is resumed. Hartmann's solution can be used, but additional potassium may be needed to bring the concentration to 20 mEq per litre of infusion fluid if the patient is vomiting or has diarrhoea. As much as five or ten litres of fluid may be required before the patient is ready for operation.

Acid-base disturbances

Metabolic acidosis will develop acutely following any event in which tissue perfusion is inadequate and tissue hypoxia, leading to anaerobic metabolism, occurs. This applies to cardiac arrest, profound hypotension, respiratory arrest and ischaemia of any part of the body (for example, when a tourniquet is applied to a limb). The clinical signs of severe metabolic acidosis are hypotension with cold, cyanosed extremities, hyperpnoea and tracheal tug, and drowsiness. Metabolic acidosis also occurs in diabetic ketosis, during very rapid blood transfusion, in renal failure and in prolonged diarrhoea. The treatment is infusion of isotonic sodium bicarbonate (1.4 per cent) which contains 1 mEq in 6 ml. In the average case 50–100 mEq will be needed to correct the acidosis, depending on the clinical signs. Recovery is associated with the metabolism of excess lactic acid in the liver, which produces further bicarbonate, so over-treatment should be avoided.

Metabolic alkalosis occurs in vomiting due to pyloric stenosis, after a treated hypoxic episode and after massive blood transfusion as the citric and lactic acids in stored blood are metabolised in the liver. The effects are underventilation, the respiratory response which raises the arterial carbon dioxide tension, and lowering of serum potassium level, which may be associated with tetany or increased muscular irritability. The urine is alkaline. The condition is better avoided than treated, but isotonic sodium chloride should be infused, to which 20 mEq potassium per litre should be added.

Blood transfusion

In some regions there is a high incidence of transfusion reactions and the routine use of antihistamines is common. In any case transfusion should only be undertaken as a routine procedure when a good laboratory with dependable workers is available; otherwise incompatibility and infection or haemolysis of blood will occur. In the absence of adequate facilities it should be used only when otherwise the patient is likely to die (Batten, 1961).

Autotransfusion is possible when patients have massive intraperitoneal or intrathoracic bleeding. The blood should have been freshly shed and there must be no likelihood of it being infected. Suitable cases are those with rupture of the liver or spleen or an ectopic gestation or with chest or pelvic injuries. The blood is removed with a ladle or sucker and strained through fine gauze into a transfusion bottle. Such blood is defibrinated and will not clot, so anticoagulant is unnecessary. It has the advantages that it will carry oxygen and that no cross matching is needed.

Exchange transfusion has been found valuable for patients with severe anaemia (haemoglobin concentration below 4 g per 100 ml blood). These patients tend to develop pulmonary oedema when given even small amounts of blood, of the order of 250 ml. Exchange transfusion of 1000 to 1500 ml results in marked clinical improvement with, for example, recovery of consciousness in a formerly comatose patient (Fullerton and Turner, 1962). The method can be used during labour or operation and is quite simple. Blood is withdrawn via a femoral vein catheter into a 2000 ml sterile calibrated bottle containing heparin, to which suction is applied. Donor blood is given via an infusion set, 3-way tap and 50 or 100 ml syringe into an arm vein. 50–100 ml of blood is withdrawn before transfusion is started and this volume deficit is maintained throughout the procedure. An accurate balance record must be kept. The blood which has been withdrawn can later be concentrated and re-infused.

Blood stored in Acid-Citrate-Dextrose solution has a pH of 6.8 when first drawn, falling to 6.4 or 6.5 after three weeks due to the formation of lactic acid by the anaerobic metabolism of the erythrocytes. During massive transfusion, unlikely to be employed in the conditions considered in this book, there is a risk of citrate intoxication causing myocardial depression. In these cases 0.5 g calcium chloride should be given with each 500 ml unit of blood. Three weeks old stored blood also has a free potassium concentration of around 20 mEq per litre and large transfusions are accompanied by the risk of myocardial depression due to hyperkalaemia. Lastly, hypothermia will develop during massive transfusion unless the blood is first passed through a warming cell.

Nevertheless, blood transfusion is an essential life-saving technique in patients with major injuries. For less severe operations careful attention to haemostasis will ensure minimal operative loss. The volume lost should be estimated by using swabs of standard size whose dry weight can be determined. Swabs are weighed after use on a 100 g spring balance. 1 ml of blood weighs 1 g. Suction bottles should be calibrated by adding known volumes of water and attaching marks (made of embossing tape) to the outside. The loss should be updated regularly and written on a board placed where the surgeon can easily see it. Losses up to 500 ml (10 per cent of the adult blood volume) can be replaced by two to three times this volume of Hartmann's solution.

Setting up a drip

It is important in patients undergoing surgery that the drip should run easily for as long as it is likely to be needed. It must permit the giving of anaesthetic and other drugs and transfusion of blood in the event of haemorrhage and must continue to function even if the patient is restless after the operation.

The site of the infusion should be carefully chosen so that the needle or cannula does not overly a joint. If possible the left arm (except in the case of a left-handed patient) should be used, so that he can use his right arm freely after the operation. The cephalic vein at the lower end of the forearm is the best site; the vein is large and lies just beneath the skin, making it easy to enter. It is possible to reduce or avoid the need for splinting the arm if this site is used, the arm itself splinting the needle.

In order to secure an open vein before the start of anaesthesia it is advisable to set up the drip under local anaesthesia. A tourniquet, consisting of a length of soft rubber tubing knotted round the arm, is applied above the elbow. This should exert just sufficient pressure to occlude the veins. The arterial supply must not be occluded or the veins will not fill, so the radial artery should be felt to check that it is pulsating. The arm is extended and allowed to rest on a firm surface. The skin should be cleaned with alcohol and the chosen vein gently patted to encourage it to dilate. Lignocaine 1 per cent is injected just distal to the estimated point of entry into the vein so as to raise the skin weal about 1 cm diameter, as illustrated in Figure 6.1.

The infusion needle or needle-cannula set is then passed through the skin weal, alongside the line of the vein. In order to prevent it entering the vein too rapidly and possibly transfixing it, the skin and the vein must be

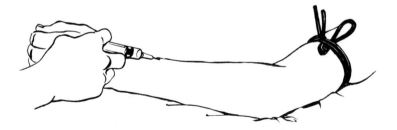

Fig. 6.1   A venous tourniquet has been applied to the arm. Local anaesthetic is being injected into the skin

entered in two separate and distinct movements. Next, the needle is manoeuvred so that its point lies over the vein. The point is then depressed so as to pucker the vein wall and the needle advanced into the vein (Figure 6.2). In the case of needle-cannula sets, the cannula is then held by the operator's free hand and advanced further up the vein while the needle is held stationary as shown in Figure 6.3. This will ensure that the tip of the cannula rests well above the point at which the vein might have been damaged by the needle tip. The skin over the tip of the cannula is then compressed with the third finger of the hand holding the cannula in order to prevent back flow of blood while the introducing needle is being withdrawn and the infusion set connected (Figure 6.4). The tubing and cannula or needle should be firmly fixed with strapping, ensuring that they lie along the line of the vein. It is a good idea to loop the tubing, as shown in Figure 6.5, to prevent the needle from being jerked out of the vein by mistake.

In a shocked patient it may be necessary to cut down on to a vein. In this case a tourniquet is applied as described above. A rather large skin weal is raised above the site of the empty vein, which can often be recognised by a trough beneath the skin. If the vein can be located in this way, a longitudinal incision is made through the skin weal. Otherwise, if a search has to be made, a transverse incision will be needed. Clear the vein from the subcutaneous tissue so that it can be lifted by the forceps. A needle-cannula unit is then carefully inserted into the exposed vein and, while the needle is held stationary, the cannula is advanced along the vein. Use of a needle-cannula set has the advantage that there is no leakage round the hole in the vein, which is expanded by the tapered cannula. There is no need to ligate the vein, so it can recannulate rapidly when the cannula is withdrawn. The skin is sutured. The hub of the cannula may also be sutured down for additional security. The tubing is connected and strapped down as described above.

The choice of needle or cannula is important. The flow through any tube depends on the head of pressure (i.e. the height of the bottle or pack),

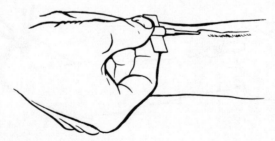

Fig. 6.2   The needle and cannula have been passed through the skin and manoeuvred so as to overlie the vein, the needle point puckering the vein wall

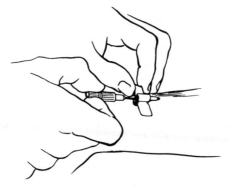

Fig. 6.3   The introducing needle is held stationary while the cannula is advanced a little way up the vein

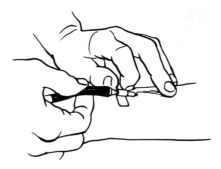

Fig. 6.4   The needle has been removed while the tip of the cannula is occluded by finger pressure. The infusion set is connected

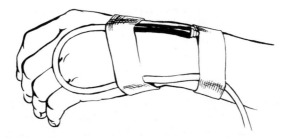

Fig. 6.5   The cannula and tubing are strapped in place. The tubing is looped so that a sudden pull is unlikely to remove the cannula

the length of the tube (as would be expected, a shorter tube passes a proportionately greater flow), and on the viscosity of the fluid (the more viscous the fluid, the slower the flow). Flow is directly proportional to the fourth power of the radius of the tube, so that doubling the radius will permit a sixteenfold increase in flow. The viscosity of stored blood is about twice that of water, and its rate of flow through any given cannula is therefore about half that of an aqueous solution. Viscosity also increases at low temperatures, being about two and a half times greater at 0°C than at 37°C. Gentle warming of blood to body temperature will not only prevent hypothermia, but will allow more rapid transfusion (Farman and Powell, 1969).

The commonest mistake is to use a long, thin needle instead of a short, wide one. The needles provided with some infusion sets are ideal, being greater than 1 mm bore and 4 cm long. These will pass blood at a reasonable rate for transfusion, but smaller sizes will prove dangerously slow. When choosing a plastic cannula, select one with thin walls, large bore (1 mm or greater for blood) and short length. The tip of the cannula should taper gently and fit tightly round the introducing needle, which should extend about 1 mm beyond it. An ideal type of cannula is shown in Figure 6.6. There is sometimes confusion over the sizing of needles and cannulae. Manufacturers vary from those who will give all possible dimensions, to the completely uninformative. British manufactures use inches or millimetres and Standard Wire Gauge (SWG), American manufacturers and their subsidiaries use inches and Standard Wire Gauge (usually shortened to 'Ga'), and Continental European manufacturers use millimetres. Table 6.2 gives equivalent sizes in these systems.

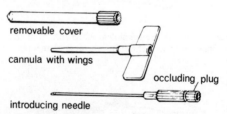

Fig. 6.6   A typical cannula.

Other preoperative measures

Before the patient is given his premedication, he should sign his consent to the operation. He will not be capable of doing this once he becomes sleepy. He should also empty his bladder; a full bladder is uncomfortable and will cause restlessness during induction and in the recovery period. False teeth, jewellery, watch, rings, hair clips, spectacles, contact lenses,

Table 6.2. Conversion Table for Standard Wire Gauge, Millimetres and Inches

SWG	mm	Inches
26	0.45	0.018
25	0.51	0.020
24	0.56	0.022
23	0.61	0.024
22	0.71	0.028
21	0.81	0.032
20	0.91	0.036
19	1.0	0.040
18	1.2	0.048
17	1.4	0.056
16	1.6	0.064
15	1.8	0.072
14	2.0	0.080
13	2.3	0.092
12	2.6	0.104
11	3.0	0.116
10	3.3	0.128

false eyes, concealed deaf aids, artificial limbs and false eyelashes should be removed; in short everything which may fall off and get broken. These objects should be put in a safe place in a paper bag marked with the patient's name. He should then get into bed to take his premedication, after which he must be allowed to rest quietly until the time of operation is due.

Whenever possible steps should be taken to ensure that the patient's stomach is empty before the induction of anaesthesia. It is usually considered necessary for him to abstain from food for four to six hours (preferably the latter) and from drink for two to four hours. The emptying time of the stomach may be prolonged in children, during labour, by anxiety and by pathological conditions (e.g. pyloric stenosis). It is never possible to guarantee that the stomach is empty. Although the use of a naso-gastric tube will be helpful in reducing intra-gastric pressure in patients with bowel obstruction, no tube can completely empty the stomach.

Premedication

This should really be considered part of the anaesthetic, as good premedication will make the anaesthetic go smoothly, but premedication of the wrong sort or at the wrong time will lead to a stormy or difficult experience for both the patient and the anaesthetist. The aims of premedication are to protect the patient from anxiety about the impending operation, to protect him from side effects of the anaesthetic and to make the induction of anaesthesia easier. Nowadays a large number of drugs is available for this purpose. When prescribing premedicants it is essential to have regard to the weight of the patient, otherwise overdosage will result. In some hospitals it may be most convenient to let the patient walk to the theatre block. In this case the premedication must not be heavy enough to cause postural hypotension (see below).

Belladonna Alkaloids

The use of atropine or hyoscine is essential in the preparation of a patient for an ether anaesthetic. These drugs have two main effects. Firstly, they prevent the excessive salivation which is a feature of ether anaesthesia, particularly when an endotracheal tube is not used. Secondly, in a large enough dose, they can also protect against bradycardia. When halothane or chloroform, which produce bradycardia, are to be used, this is an important consideration. However, this is not a danger in ether anaesthesia in which the heart rate is usually within the normal range. The use of atropine is associated with an appreciable (27 per cent) incidence of cardiac arrhythmias when intubation with suxamethonium is employed, whereas the incidence when hyoscine is used is negligible (2 per cent) (Hart and Bryce-Smith, 1963). Small doses of atropine and moderate doses of hyoscine cause bradycardia and a large dose must be used if an increase in heart rate is desired. Atropine has no important central nervous system effects, but hyoscine produces sedation and amnesia which are useful in premedication. The dose of these drugs is 0.01 mg per kg so that the average adult will receive 0.5 to 0.75 mg of either drug. Children are given larger doses of atropine on a weight basis. However, care should be taken when using atropine for children in a hot, dry atmosphere because sweating is inhibitied and hyperpyrexia and convulsions may result. Old people do not tolerate very large doses of hyoscine, which may cause mental confusion and disorientation, and the dose should be reduced for them. These drugs can be given either orally or intramuscularly.

Opioids

These include morphine, papaveretum, pethidine,and the many other drugs in this class. They all have in common the ability to depress respiration and are therefore contra-indicated before ether anaesthesia unless the patient actually has pain. The reason for this is that the uptake of ether depends on the volume of respiration and the use of opioids will tend to slow induction of ether anaesthesia. Patients premedicated with these drugs develop low arterial oxygen tension under ether/air anaesthesia (Markello and King, 1964; Marshall and Grange, 1966). The use of opioids in premedication increases the incidence of post-operative vomiting (Dundee et al., 1965). In the case of patients who are in pain, sufficient analgesic should be given to control the pain and to prevent the patient becoming excited during the induction. More than this will depress respiration. To quote Guedel (1937), 'The employment of a routine dose of morphine is folly.'

Sedatives and tranquillisers

There are many new additions to this group of drugs, some of which are very useful in preparing patients for ether anaesthesia. Diazepam, 0.5 mg per kg orally and chlordiazepoxide, 2 mg per kg orally, induce sedation, relief of anxiety and amnesia for the pre-operative period. They are relatively non-toxic and in the doses recommended do not depress respiration. Other tranquillisers may prove equally useful but these two have been most widely used for this purpose. Barbiturates are not satisfactory before ether anaesthesia because in large doses they depress respiration and they tend to cause post-operative restlessness and disorientation.

Another extremely useful drug is Droperidol, which is given in a dose of 0.2 mg per kg intramuscularly or 0.4 mg per kg orally. It acts as a 'pharmacological restraining strap', making the patient lie still and preventing the expression of excitement. Although patients who are given this drug may appear to be heavily sedated, they have no subjective feeling of tranquillity whatsoever. Indeed they may suffer from exaggerated fears of the operation and it should therefore never be used alone for premedication, but should be accompanied by a true sedative such as diazepam. It is used for patients in whom post-operative restlessness may endanger the success of the operation, such as those having ophthalmic or plastic operations.

Route of administration

Premedication for routine operations can conveniently be given by mouth two hours before operation. The advantages of oral premedication are:

1) The drugs do not have to be drawn up into a syringe but can be given in the form of tablets
2) It is pleasanter for the patient
3) Drugs given by mouth are absorbed comparatively slowly, so the duration of action is longer and the timing needs to be less exact.

A minimal quantity of water may be given at this time.

When the patient is thought to have a full stomach or is to undergo an abdominal operation, drugs should be given by intramuscular injection one hour beforehand. In emergencies is it safer and easier to give intravenous atropine only, immediately before the induction of anaesthesia.

The anaesthetic room

For any hospital in which an appreciable number of operations is performed
it is best to have a room separate from the operating theatre to use for the
induction of anaesthesia. This room should be large enough to take the
patient on his bed or trolley, together with all the anaesthetic equipment. It
should have large doors at either end; one end should lead directly into
the theatre via a door with a small observation window. Ideally it should
be fitted with adequate concealed lighting (to avoid dazzling the patient)
and an adjustable wall lamp. It should have a sink and a large bench for
cleaning and preparing apparatus and drawing-up drugs, efficient suction
apparatus and a stand for oxygen cylinders. Cupboards, drawers and shelves
are needed for storing drugs, anaesthetic apparatus and sterile equipment
such as needles, syringes and infusion sets.

There are many advantages in having an anaesthetic room. Firstly, the
patient need not see the interior of the theatre itself and he can wait for
his operation without being disturbed. Secondly, the anaesthetist can
proceed with the induction of anaesthesia, setting up a drip and so on,
while the theatre is being prepared for the operation, in the knowledge
that all his equipment is within reach. Lastly, the anaesthetic room is a
useful centre for storing and preparing drugs and infusions for the theatre.
On the other hand, in a small hospital where the doctor must supervise
all the theatre activities, it will undoubtedly be safer to bring the patient
into the theatre before the start of the anaesthetic.

When the patient arrives it is essential to check his identity (by asking
him his name, not by saying 'are you Mr. So-and-so?'), and that he has
had his premedication at the correct time. Check that he has consented
to the operation and that operation to which he has consented is the
correct one (e.g. left inguinal herniorrhaphy as opposed to right). Once
he is asleep it will be too late to ask. It is often convenient to do such
things as shaving the patient's skin, changing blankets, etc. in the
anaesthetic room. Then a blood pressure cuff and stethoscope should be
placed on the patient's arm and the blood pressure taken and recorded on
the anaesthetic record sheet. This reading can later be compared with
those taken during the course of the anaesthetic. If an intravenous drip
or indwelling venous needle is to be used, it can be placed in the vein.
The patient will then be ready for the anaesthetic to begin.

Anaesthetic records

The act of rendering a patient unconscious is of sufficient importance to
require that a record be kept of it in the notes. This should include the
doses of drugs, fluid infused and the procedure followed, including such
details as the size of endotracheal tube used. Any untoward reactions

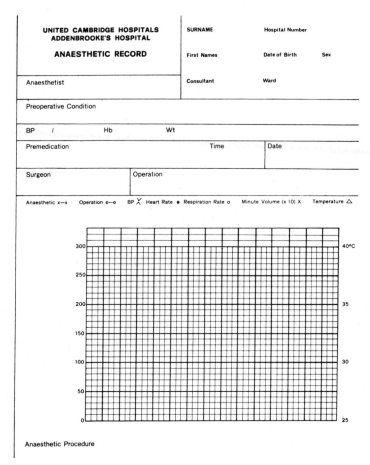

Fig. 6.7   Anaesthetic record chart

should also be noted so that they can be avoided during any subsequent anaesthetic. It is best to use a specially printed sheet with a graph for recording blood pressure, heart rate, etc. An example is shown in Figure 6.7. Complete and accurate records of anaesthetics are important, not only for individual cases but as an aid to understanding and for legal reasons in case any doubt should arise about the conduct of the anaesthetic.

Setting up the apparatus

As mentioned in Chapter 1, it is possible to combine the vaporisers, bellows, valves and other components in a variety of ways to suit individual circumstances. Certain principles must be observed if the most efficient arrangement is to be achieved.

1) If vaporisers are to be placed in series, that for the more volatile agent should be placed upstream (i.e. further from the patient) from the vaporiser for the less volatile. If this point is neglected, condensation of the less volatile agent (which will have a lower boiling point) will occur in a cooler downstream vaporiser. The E.M.O. should therefore always be upstream of the O.M.V. or B.S.I.U. (which can only be fitted on the outlet of the E.M.O. in any case). When using serial O.M.V.s for halothane and trichloroethylene, the halothane O.M.V. should be upstream.

2) The bellows or inflating bag should be placed between the vaporiser and the patient. If air is blown through the vaporiser, the concentration delivered may be greater than indicated (see Chapter 4). The E.M.O. is particularly affected by this because of its large internal volume. Parkhouse (1966) suggests that the O.M.V. will not be so affected, but it is nevertheless preferable to keep the vaporiser upstream. The exception is that when the P.B.U. is used with the E.M.O. and O.M.V. or B.S.I.U., the bellows should be placed between the two vaporisers to avoid overbalancing them.

3) Oxygen and nitrous oxide (when used) should always be introduced on the upstream side of the vaporisers. This avoids the dilution of the vapour which will occur if the gas is introduced downstream. The oxygen inlets on the O.I.B. and P.B.U. are only intended for use in resuscitation.

4) When using the O.I.B. the magnet must be used to immobilise the downstream flap valve whenever an automatic non-rebreathing valve is used. This valve must not be immobilised if a simple spring-loaded expiratory valve is used (see Chapter 4).

5) Before using the apparatus to anaesthetise a patient, the bag or bellows must be operated in order to ensure that the flow of air is in the correct direction (i.e. towards the patient).

The actual arrangement preferred will depend on the technique to be employed and on the circumstances in which it is to be used. For permanent use in a hospital the E.M.O. will form the basis of the system, taking advantage of the economy and safety of ether. It will be most convenient to mount the apparatus on a small trolley which can also support the O.I.B., laryngoscope, tubes, airways, sphygmomanometer and so on. The specially built Hospital Stand is, of course, designed for this very purpose. Regulators and rotameters for gases can be fixed to this stand. With the addition of an O.M.V., such a machine provides the same facilities as a conventional gas machine, with the additional advantage that it is not totally dependent on medical gases or the more expensive inhalational agents.

If it is necessary to move the equipment around (from hospital to hospital, for example), the Penlon Portable Outfit, consisting of the E.M.O., P.B.U., and Ambu Valve, is the most suitable arrangement. The makers provide a carrying case which has room for most of the necessary accessories, including an O.M.V. or B.S.I.U. This can easily be carried by car, but is rather too heavy (about 10 kg) for convenient hand carriage.

For the utmost in portability the combination of one or two O.M.V. s with the Aga Polyvalve Anestor is the best. Even with all the accessory equipment, the total weight will be less than half that of the E.M.O. alone. This is particularly suitable for the expert anaesthetist who is capable of employing a relaxant technique with artificial respiration, which requires very little of the inhalation agent (see Chapter 9).

Figure 6.8 shows the various ways in which the component parts of the system can be combined.

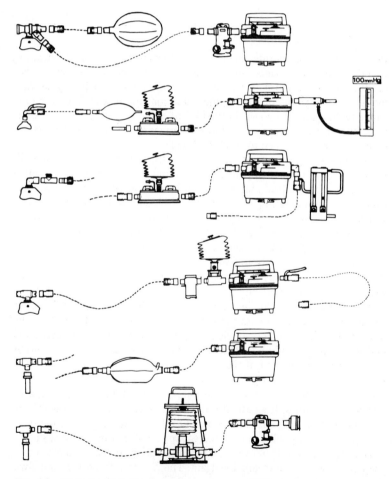

Fig. 6.8   Ways in which the apparatus can be assembled

Chapter Seven

Induction Techniques

It is convenient to consider the conduct of anaesthesia under the headings of induction, maintenance and the end of anaesthesia. Various methods of producing unconsciousness can be employed, each of which may be followed by different ways of completing the induction and by a variety of maintenance techniques. Moreover, in the case of ether, a well-defined procedure must be followed before surgical anaesthesia is attained. This chapter describes the steps taken to reach this stage.

Before starting the anaesthetic, the anaesthetist should ensure that all the necessary drugs and apparatus are to hand, the equipment for dealing with complications (suction, oxygen, intubation equipment, intravenous fluids and administration sets) is within reach and that all apparatus is working. The danger to the patient's life, from respiratory obstruction, vomiting or circulatory depression is greatest during the period of induction. The utmost skill and attention should be available at this time.

Patients who are likely to vomit, that is children, women in labour, patients with bowel obstruction and any emergency, provide the anaesthetist with his most worrying times. The steps described here should never be omitted. For the inexperienced anaesthetist it is best to employ an inhalation induction with the patient lying on his side. It will be found quite easy to keep the airway clear in this position. The pharyngeal suction end should be pushed under the pillow while an assistant should stand by in order to raise the foot of the trolley immediately the anaesthetist gives the word. Vomiting is triggered off by respiratory obstruction and by unsuccessful attempts at artificial respiration, which inflate the stomach instead of the lungs. If a patient does vomit during induction, the foot of the trolley should be raised immediately. The second step is the use of suction. The lungs will be protected against inhaled vomitus by laryngeal spasm, but this results in hypoxia. When the pharynx has been cleared the patient will begin to breathe again. The first few breaths should always be enriched with oxygen.

1) *Producing unconsciousness*

a)   *With ether*

The simplest, but in many ways the most tedious method of induction, is by the use of ether and air alone. Because the E.M.O. gives known concentrations of ether, it is possible to increase the inspired concentration in a much smoother and more controllable manner than with the open drop method. It will be found that the most a conscious patient can breathe is 3 or 4 per cent and this concentration is therefore used to start with. In a co-operative patient the mask may be placed directly on the face to obtain an airtight fit. In children and nervous adults it is better to hold the mask a few centimetres above the face and to work the bellows up and down so as to pump the ether/air mixture towards the patient until he shows signs of going to sleep, when the mask can be placed directly on the face. This method, of course, takes more time. It is essential for successful inhalational induction both to maintain a perfect airway and to obtain a good fit of the mask, as described in Chapter 5, to ensure that the patient breathes only the anaesthetic mixture. The best type of mask will depend on the shape of the face of the patient. Once a good fit has been obtained, the concentration of ether is increased by 1 per cent about every 4 breaths until consciousness is lost, as shown by the loss of the eyelash reflex. The first stage of ether anaesthesia is referred to as the stage of analgesia, which is detectable even before consciousness is lost. The achievement of surgical anaesthesia is described in section 2 of this chapter.

b)   *With intravenous agents*

The use of intravenous agents to produce unconsciousness can make induction both quicker and pleasanter for the patient. The most commonly used agent is thiopentone, although other agents may also be used. Very short acting drugs, such as methohexitone and propanidid, are less suitable because their effects wear off very quickly. The following description therefore applies to the use of 2.5 per cent thiopentone. The dose needed for producing unconsciousness will be of the order of 5 mg per kg. In other words, it is nearly always less than 0.5 g and usually about 200–300 mg. This will be enough to make the patient go off to sleep for a few minutes only. As soon as he is asleep, the mask is applied and he is allowed to breathe 3–4 per cent ether in air. Patients frequently take a few deep breaths, followed by a short period of apnoea. This is seldom sufficiently prolonged to require artificial respiration provided that no morphine or other respiratory depressant has been given. Allowance should be made for the unusually slow circulation times found in patients with low cardiac outputs. Overdosage with thiopentone will depress both respiration and circulation. In oligaemia a normal dose of the drug will mix with a small volume of blood, achieving an abnormally high concentration. This will exacerbate its cardiovascular effect, sometimes producing a precipitous fall in arterial pressure, which should be treated by raising the foot of the table or trolley 5–10 degrees, giving the patient 100 per cent oxygen and running in 500 ml of electrolyte solution. If the heart rate is slow, 0.25 mg atropine should be given intravenously. If the pressure fails to rise, give the patient 100 mg calcium chloride. However, this complication is better avoided by ensuring adequate pre-operative treatment of oligaemia. Induction then proceeds to the stage of surgical anaesthesia as described in section 2 below.

For minor procedures such as incising an abscess or reducing a Colles fracture, anaesthesia can be produced with thiopentone alone. It is essential for all preparations for the operation to be made before the injection is given, including cleaning the skin and placing of towels. About 5 mg/kg is then injected in the way described below. The needle is kept in the vein and as soon as consciousness is lost the head is extended in order to ensure a clear airway. The jaw is supported by an assistant if necessary. The surgeon must do the operation immediately, before the peak effect of the drug wears off. If the patient moves, a further 50–100 mg is given. In emergencies, longer operations can be performed under this form of anaesthesia. The disadvantage is that the patient may remain sedated for many hours afterwards. For regular use of this method it would be better to employ methohexitone or propanidid which have fewer after effects.

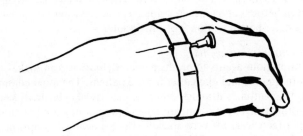

Fig. 7.1   Gordh diaphragm needle in place

A vein is selected on the lateral side of the cubital fossa or the back of the hand. The back of the hand is chosen for insertion of an indwelling self-sealing needle such as the Gordh (Figure 7.1) or Mitchell types. This method is recommended if more than one injection is likely to be needed (e.g. when a relaxant is to be used), but when an intravenous infusion is not used. However, the soft rubber segment of a drip set permits repeated injections and allows an infusion to take the place of a self-sealing needle. For direct intravenous injection a venous tourniquet is applied (a piece of rubber tubing lightly knotted round the arm or the hand of an assistant applying gentle pressure above the level of the vein). It is important not to apply so much pressure that the arterial supply to the limb is occluded, otherwise the veins will never fill and it will be impossible to tell an artery from a vein. Great care must be taken to avoid injecting into an artery, so the vessel is palpated to ensure that it is not pulsating. The skin at the site of venepuncture is cleaned with spirit (alcohol) and the vein is gently patted with the fingers to make it dilate. The needle is then inserted into the skin, pointing up the arm immediately lateral to the vein. As soon as the point is through the skin, it is manoeuvred sideways until it lies over the vein. The point is then depressed so as to pucker the vein wall. It is then advanced into the vein and an aspiration test made, as shown in Figure 7.2. If this shows that the needle is within the vein, the assistant relaxes his grip or the tourniquet is removed. The syringe and needle should be laid alongside the arm or flat against the back of the hand and the hub gripped with the thumb of one hand while the fingers extend around the limb. A small quantity (2 ml) of the intravenous agent is injected and the patient is asked whether his arm is comfortable. If he says that he is

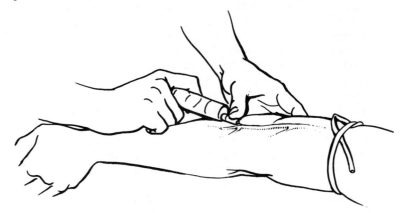

Fig. 7.2   Induction with thiopentone. The tourniquet should in fact be removed before the injection is made. Note that a vein on the *lateral* aspect of the cubital fossa is used

comfortable, the remainder of the dose can be given slowly. If pain follows, it suggests that the injection has been made into an artery. If this happens the limb will blanch and the distal pulses will become impalpable due to intravascular crystalisation of the drug (Waters, 1966). The treatment is to leave the needle in the vessel, but remove the syringe and inject through the needle 5 ml of 2 per cent procaine or lignocaine to dilate the vessel. Local anaesthetic solution is then infiltrated around the vessel in order to block the sympathetic nerve supply. The risk of serious consequences (e.g. gangrene of a hand) is greatly reduced when 2.5 per cent, as opposed to 5 per cent, thiopentone is used.

c)   With an accessory vaporiser

The Oxford Miniature Vaporiser (O.M.V.) was originally designed to assist
in induction of ether anaesthesia by using halothane (Parkhouse, 1966).
Respiratory tract reflexes are profoundly depressed by halothane, making
it an almost ideal agent for this purpose (Holmes and Bryce-Smith, 1964).
The O.M.V. fits the outlet of the E.M.O. When using the Penlon Bellows
(P.B.U.) it is easier to fit the bellows directly to the E.M.O., followed by
the O.M.V. on the patient's side of the P.B.U. This does not affect the
performance of the vaporiser and prevents the whole unit over-balancing
when the bellows is used. The vaporiser is filled with 10 ml halothane
and the mask placed on the patient's face. The halothane concentration is
turned to 1 per cent and the patient allowed to breathe this mixture. The
ether concentration is turned to 3—4 per cent. The patient will go off to
sleep very quickly and as he does so the ether concentration is increased
steadily to 20 per cent. It will be found that this can be done very much
more quickly than when ether is used on its own, taking less than 10 minutes, even for a large man. The incidence of coughing, breath-holding and
laryngeal spasm is reduced by using halothane (Markello and King, 1964).
The halothane must be left on the 1 per cent setting until 15—20 per cent
ether has been reached. If surgical anaesthesia has not been achieved
by this time, then halothane may be continued until this has happened. If
more than 1 per cent halothane is used the patient's blood pressure is
likely to fall alarmingly. For this reason the blood pressure should be
taken every 3 to 4 minutes during the induction period. Figure 7.3 shows
that some fall in arterial pressure is the rule during this type of induction.
Exposure to the combination of 1 per cent halothane and 15—20 per cent
ether will eventually depress even the circulation of a fit, healthy subject,
as illustrated in Figure 7.4. In shocked patients it is recommended that
not more than 0.5 per cent halothane be used, which will normally be
found sufficient for these subjects. Higher concentrations of halothane may
also depress respiration but 1 per cent vapour does not prevent the
increase in ventilation which normally follows the use of ether, as shown
in Figure 7.5.

For short cases, such as opening abscesses and reduction of Colles'
fractures, it is permissable to give a higher concentration of halothane, up
to 2—3 per cent, as the sole anaesthetic agent. This will cost no more than
using thiopentone, but has the advantage that it is more controllable,
particularly if the operation goes on for a few minutes longer than
anticipated. Oxygen 2 litres per minute should be added to the inspired
mixture because of the risk of respiratory depression.

It is also possible to use the O.M.V. for trichloroethylene and in this
case 1 per cent should be set on the vaporiser. Trichloroethylene is a less
powerful narcotic than halothane and the induction may therefore take
rather longer. However, it is a cheap and useful way of assisting ether

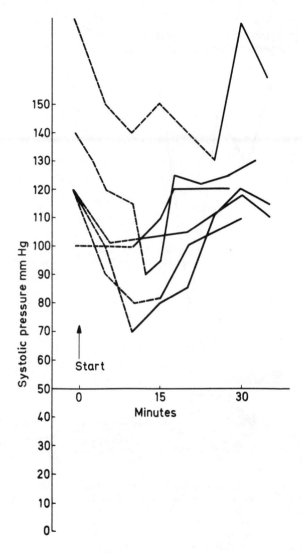

Fig. 7.3   Effect of 1 per cent halothane during induction. Systolic pressure in six patients given 1 per cent halothane with the O.M.V. (dotted lines). All continued to breathe 15 or 20 per cent ether after the halothane was turned off (solid lines)

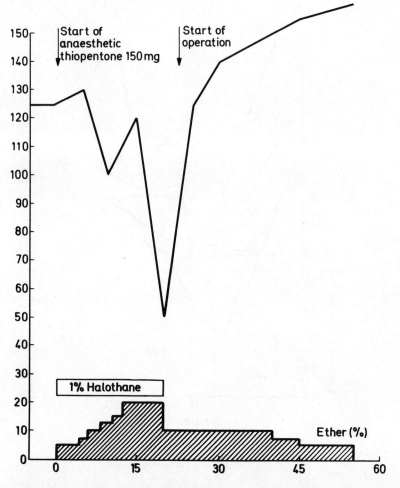

Fig. 7.4   Sudden fall in systolic arterial pressure 20 minutes after the start of anaesthesia, accompanied by cyanosis and apnoea. 1 per cent halothane was being given from an O.M.V. in series with the E.M.O. The halothane was turned off and the ether concentration reduced to 10 per cent. Artificial respiration with oxygen was given for half a minute, but when the operation began the patient started to breathe again and the blood pressure returned to normal

induction (Tunstall, 1963). It is safer than halothane for seriously ill patients and for children. The combined use of halothane and trichloroethylene is described in Chapter 8.

The Bryce-Smith Induction Unit (Bryce-Smith, 1963) is also designed

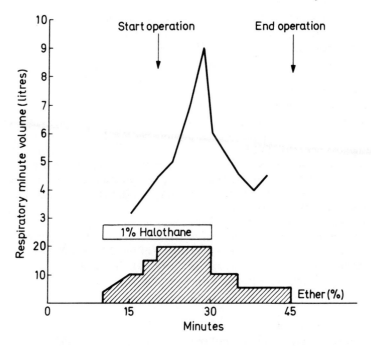

Fig. 7.5   Change in respiratory minute volume (litres) during induction with ether and 1 per cent halothane, using the E.M.O. and O.M.V. in series

for halothane. It is filled as described earlier (see Chapter 4) and attached to the outlet of the E.M.O. When the P.B.U. is used, it should be fitted on the patient side of the bellows. The dose is limited to 3 ml for safety reasons; little respiratory or cardiac depression results in adults, making it suitable for relatively unskilled administrators. The cost of 3 ml halothane is only about 5p, making it cheaper than 0.5 g thiopentone. The ether concentration is set to 3–4 per cent before the mask is placed on the patient's face. Obviously an absolutely airtight fit is essential. As soon as the patient starts to breathe through the mask, he will inhale the halothane which achieves a concentration of about 3 per cent, but only for 3 or 4 minutes before the supply is exhausted. This means that for a short while the concentration delivered is greater than with the O.M.V. (used as described above), but is less long lasting. The idea is to increase the concentration of ether very rapidly, in steps of 2 per cent every 4–5 breaths, to 15–20 per cent (Holmes and Bryce-Smith, 1964). It should take 2–4.5 minutes to reach this concentration and between 4.5 and 15 minutes before a tube can be passed. It will be found that while it works well for large children and small women, it is less satisfactory for robust adult males, who tend to wake up before the ether concentration can be increased sufficiently. A small fall of arterial pressure is common, often accompanied by dysrhythmia, especially on laryngoscopy and intubation. The unit can also be used with trichloroethylene, a method recommended for children (see Chapter 10) and with chloroform.

Both the O.M.V. and the Bryce-Smith Induction Unit can be used for providing inhalational analgesia with trichloroethylene or methoxyflurane. The O.M.V. is more suitable for this purpose because the effect is longer lasting. 0.5 per cent of either agent is required. A facemask and non-rebreathing valve are connected to the vaporiser by a length of corrugated tubing. No bellows is needed. This is useful in labour and for the dressing of burns, during painful physiotherapy and for changes of dressings and manipulation of fractures.

A home-made accessory vaporiser, consisting of an angle-piece and an inverted facemask covered with gauze, has been described (Bhardwaj and Coghlan, 1965). This is fitted to the air inlet of the E.M.O. and 3—4 ml halothane dropped onto the gauze from a (glass) syringe during induction. The use of divinyl ether from a dropper unit in series with the E.M.O. is also a possibility.

d)   With ketamine

This drug can be used for the intravenous induction of anaesthesia or as the sole anaesthetic for minor procedures. However it is rather too expensive for routine use as an induction agent. It is also effective after intramuscular injection, which is the route of choice in restless or unco-operative patients. 5 mg/kg will induce a state of drowsiness in 3—5 minutes, lasting 15—30 minutes, after which anaesthesia may be continued and made deeper with inhalational agents. The intravenous dose is around 2 mg/kg, administered slowly to avoid respiratory depression, which produces 5—10 minutes anaesthesia, long enough to permit induction of full surgical anaesthesia with ether.

The main use of ketamine is for the performance of superficial operations and painful diagnostic procedures. Examples are painful endoscopies, biopsies, dental operations, skin grafts, obstetric procedures, manipulation of fractures, redressing of wounds, and suturing of lacerations. The dose needed for this purpose is around 10 mg/kg, given by intramuscular injection. Muscle tone is retained during ketamine anaesthesia; indeed it may increase to the point of clonus or involuntary movement, so abdominal operations cannot be performed. Nystagmus may occur. Heart rate and arterial pressure commonly increase, while intra-ocular and intracranial pressures also rise, making ketamine unsuitable for patients in whom these pressures are already raised. Careful observation is therefore needed throughout operation, even though respiratory obstruction is rare. Post-operative hallucinations must be treated by giving moderate doses of tranquilliser such as diazepam. This has the advantage that the patient then remains sleepy for some hours afterwards.

2) *Attaining surgical anaesthesia*

a)   With ether
Unconsciousness will have been produced by one of the methods described above and the patient will be breathing 5–10 per cent ether by this time. If he coughs or holds his breath, then no further increase in concentration should be given until respiration is smooth again. Increments of 1 per cent are given until 10 per cent is reached, after which they are increased to 2.5 per cent. It is a good rule to allow four unobstructed breaths before increasing the concentration. The concentration can be increased to 20 per cent in healthy subjects, but severely ill patients should be limited to 10 or 15 per cent.

High concentrations of ether will depress the myocardium and when air is the carrier gas, they will reduce the oxygen concentration in the inspired mixture. For example, when the ether concentration is 20 per cent, the mixture will contain only 16 per cent oxygen. The induction time will vary with the body weight, a heavy body taking much longer to become saturated than a light one; similarly excretion takes longer in a heavy person. During induction, a larger quantity of ether is usually consumed than for the whole of the rest of the anaesthetic, varying from 50 ml for a child to 150 ml for a man. Early on, but after attaining surgical anaesthesia, non-nervous body tissue such as muscle, fat and liver, are still absorbing ether and the inspired concentration must be kept high, but as these tissues approach saturation less and less ether has to be added in order to maintain an arterial (and hence brain) level sufficient to keep the patient anaesthetised.

Complications are likely to occur during the 'second' stage, particularly if the concentration is increased too rapidly. This stage is often described as the stage of excitement or delirium in which cortical inhibition is absent and uncontrolled reflex activity takes place. Muscle tone is increased and the eyes move from side to side ('roving'). The patient may also move his arms and legs and even attempt to get off the bed. For this reason it is absolutely essential to have an assistant standing by in order to restrain the patient at this stage. It is highly dangerous to attempt to anaesthetise a patient with ether in the absence of an assistant.

The onset of surgical anaesthesia is heralded by smooth, even respiration ('automatic respiration') and by absence of spontaneous movement of the limbs. Automatic respiration may appear during the second stage and the anaesthetist must not be misled by this. The inspired concentration is no guide to the depth of anaesthesia, high concentrations being tolerated early by some patients (Bhardwaj and Coghlan, 1965). The eyes look straight ahead in surgical anaesthesia and at first the pupils are small. The abdominal recti no longer contract with expiration and the limb muscles also relax. At this stage it is safe for the operation to start. The signs of ether anaesthesia are described in Chapter 8 (Table 8.1, page127).

Poor risk patients will not stand high concentrations of anaesthetics. Extra patience is needed because induction cannot be hurried. In patients who are likely to vomit, such as those with intestinal obstruction, induction should be purely inhalational unless a skilled anaesthetist is in charge. In shocked patients and those with chest disease or cyanosis, oxygen should be added to the inspired mixture at the rate of 2 litres per minute. This will increase the inspired oxygen concentration to approximately 40 per cent, but it will render the ether mixture explosive. Coughing, straining, and laryngeal spasm will increase the likelihood of vomiting and it will be safer to have the patient lying on his side. If vomiting occurs unexpectedly, the patient should be turned immediately onto his side and the foot of the trolley or table raised. Suction apparatus should always be at hand during induction.

While this method of induction is reliable, it does take rather a long time. It will take 15—20 minutes to bring the average man to surgical anaesthesia, 10—15 minutes for a woman and 5—10 minutes for a child. It is possible to make induction a little quicker by assisting each breath with the bellows (Farman, 1961). This can only be done if an automatic non-rebreathing valve is used. The technique consists of keeping one hand on the bellows and each time the patient inspires the breath is augmented with the bellows. During very light anaesthesia this may make the patient cough, but later on during induction it can be very useful. However, the rate and depth of respiration will usually increase automatically during an ether induction and the minute volume will often reach 15 or 20 litres or more (see Figure 7.6). If nitrous oxide is available, the ether can be vaporised in 70 per cent nitrous oxide in oxygen until surgical anaesthesia is achieved. This will also save time. The addition of 5 per cent carbon dioxide to the inspired mixture will increase alveolar ventilation and has the additional advantage of also increasing cerebral blood-flow and hence of accelerating the rate of uptake of ether by the brain (Kety, 1951). However, the advantage of these methods is not great and probably not worh the complication of the additional apparatus required.

b)   *With a relaxant and intubation*

The quickest method of induction is by the use of an intravenous agent (described above) followed by a short acting muscle relaxant such as suxamethonium. It is essential that the anaesthetist be skilled in intubation· before this method is attempted, because failure to pass a tube can result in severe anoxia and possibly death if the patient has not been pre-oxygen-

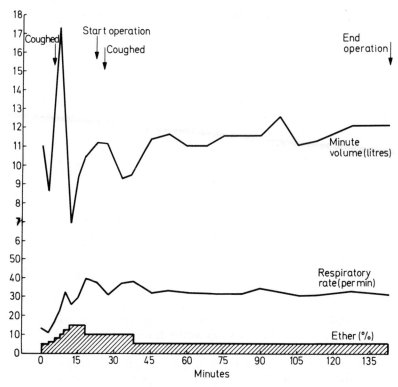

Fig. 7.6   Record of minute volume and respiratory rate in a 53 year old man having a bilateral inguinal herniorrhaphy. Note hyperventilation during the induction period. Anaesthesia with ether in air after hyoscine premedication

ated. If he is uncertain of his ability to pass a tube, he should restrict himself to intubating only under surgical anaesthesia with ether until he is fully proficient (Francis-Lau, 1964). The patient is given 100 per cent oxygen to breathe for 2–3 minutes before the injection is made. This ensures that his lungs are full of oxygen during the period of 2–3 minutes when he is paralysed by the relaxant (see Chapter 2). Thiopentone 5 mg per kg is followed immediately by suxamethonium 1 mg per kg (about 50 mg for an average adult). When it is given immediately following thiopentone, the fasciculation caused by the relaxant will appear in 15–30 seconds, and it will then be possible to pass an endotracheal tube, as described in Chapter 5. The recommended dose of suxamethonium will produce only a limited duration of paralysis in the average patient so that the action of the relaxant wears off and the patient will start to breathe again before arterial desaturation is likely to occur. For most cases the larynx and trachea should be sprayed with lignocaine 1 mg per kg, which will facilitate the smooth resumption of spontaneous respiration (see Chapter 5).

As soon as the tube has been passed the cuff is inflated, using only enough air to prevent leakage when the bellows is compressed, and the tube is fixed securely in place. The catheter mount, vapour condenser and non-rebreathing valve are connected and the ether concentration turned to 15 per cent. Artificial respiration is then carried out for a few minutes until a sufficient quantity of ether has been absorbed to prevent the patient coughing when spontaneous respiration returns. A common mistake is to fail to introduce enough ether into the patient during this period. It is essential to keep a finger on the patient's pulse when he is being ventilated with this strong concentration of ether, which may lower the cardiac output; there will be a fall of blood pressure and the pulse will become weaker An example of this is shown in Figure 7.7. Arrhythmias are common in patients premedicated with atropine (Hart and Bryce-Smith, 1963). If these complications occur the artificial respiration should be slowed, the ether concentration reduced to 10 per cent and the head end of the table tilted downwards. The blood pressure should be checked to ensure that it is not still low. After standing in a hot atmosphere, the ether chamber of the E.M.O. may contain a dangerously high concentration of vapour (up to 35 per cent) which will be delivered to the patient when it is first turned on. This concentration will cause marked cardiovascular depression, especially in an artificially ventilated patient. However, if 15 per cent is the maximum used, then the majority of patients will not suffer any serious fall of blood pressure. In very ill or shocked patients the concentration must be limited to 10 per cent. This whole procedure can be completed in under 5 minutes, a considerable saving of time in a busy operating theatre. Some difficulty may be encountered in getting the patient to breathe again, but if artificial respiration is limited to 3—4 minutes, then the patient will usually start to breathe within 15—30 seconds. If insufficient ether has been introduced the patient will cough and hold his breath and artificial respiration must be resumed for one or two minutes more before he is allowed to breathe spontaneously again. With practice it is usually possible to judge the timing correctly. The patient is allowed to breathe 15—20 per cent ether until surgical anaesthesia has been achieved.

This method has the considerable advantage for the single-handed operator that once he has passed the tube and settled the patient, he can safely hand over to a nurse who will then control the ether concentration as required. There is little danger that the airway will become obstructed, although the possibility of the tube becoming kinked must never be forgotten. It is the method of choice for the skilled intubator dealing with

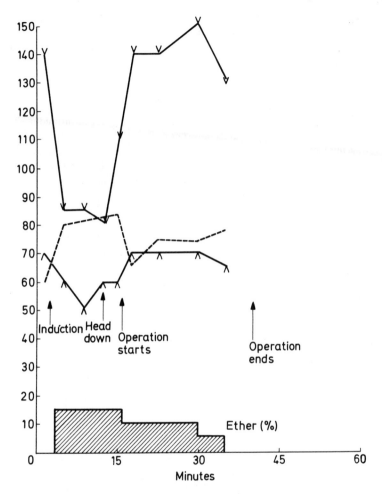

Fig. 7.7   Heart rate and arterial pressure during anaesthesia. Record of heart rate (– beats per min.) and arterial pressure (vʌmm Hg) in a 19 year old man. Anaesthesia was induced with 300 mg thiopentone followed by 50 mg suxamethonium to assist endotracheal intubation. Artificial respiration with 15 per cent ether in air was given for about 5 minutes, until spontaneous respiration returned. This was associated with hypotension and an increase in heart rate

the patient who is likely to vomit. In these cases the patient lies supine, while the assistant applies pressure over the cricoid cartilage, preventing reflux up the oesophagus, until the tube is in place and the cuff inflated. The anaesthetist attaches a full 10 ml syringe to the endotracheal cuff. As soon as the relaxant starts to work, he inserts the laryngoscope and passes the tube, which should be well lubricated. It is safer to pass a rather small tube and to be sure of getting it in than to risk being unable to insert it. As soon as it is in place the cuff is inflated. Suction should be available and the assistant should be prepared to turn the patient on his side if the patient subsequently regurgitates.

The expert anaesthetist who intends to maintain anaesthesia with the help of a longer-acting muscle relaxant (see Chapter 8) may pass the tube with the help of tubocurarine or pancuronium and proceed immediately to ventilate the lungs with a maintenance concentration of anaesthetic. Long-acting relaxants act rather less rapidly than the depolarisers and it will be necessary to ventilate the lungs for 2 or 3 minutes with an oxygen-rich mixture via a facemask before intubating (see also Chapter 8).

Chapter Eight

Maintenance of Anaesthesia

Maintenance of anaesthesia means keeping the patient in a state of surgical anaesthesia for the duration of an operation. For most purposes only ether is needed to maintain anaesthesia, but for some operations, particularly in the upper abdomen, ether alone will not provide safe muscular relaxation and other means of relaxing the abdominal muscles must be used. For operations within the chest or in the face-down position, artificial respiration will be needed and this will mean using muscle relaxants.

The use of ether for maintenance of anaesthesia

At the end of the induction period the patient will have reached the stage of surgical anaesthesia. He will normally be breathing 15 or 20 per cent ether. Because of the high solubility and comparatively low potency of ether, a considerable mass of the anaesthetic must be taken up by the body in order to achieve anaesthesia. It is usually necessary to keep the concentration control at this high concentration for 5–15 minutes, depending on the size of the patient (large patients absorb more ether) and on his general condition. It is a common mistake to reduce the concentration before the start of the operation, with the result that the patient is found to be too lightly anaesthetised when the incision is made. The concentration may be reduced to 10 per cent once it is certain that surgical anaesthesia has been properly established (the signs of anaesthesia are described below). This is maintained for a further 15–30 minutes in the average case before being finally reduced to about 5 per cent for the remainder of the operation. One of the commonest mistakes with ether is to try to use too little once the patient appears to be settled (Cole and Parkhouse, 1963). It is not often possible to reduce the maintenance concentration below 5 per cent, except towards the end of prolonged operations, and very rarely below 3 or 4 per cent, which is the equilibrium concentration for surgical anaesthesia. The consumption of ether will usually be between 2 and 2.5 ml per minute (after induction with the aid of thiopentone) but will of course vary with the size of the patient and the depth of anaesthesia.

Signs of ether anaesthesia

Although it is easy to describe a rule of thumb for giving an anaesthetic, successful management can only be achieved by an understanding of the signs of anaesthesia. In surgical anaesthesia the patient lies still under the knife, breathing is even and regular (automatic respiration), the eyes look straight ahead and at first the pupils are small and reactive, but as anaesthesia deepens, the pupils become larger and the light reaction is lost.

The size of the pupils will be influenced by the use of atropine or nitrous oxide (Cullen et al., 1972), which both dilate the pupils or by opioids given before operation, which constrict them.

The most important and reliable sign of ether anaesthesia is provided by the tone of the abdominal and thoracic muscles. During light anaesthesia the whole thorax expands during inspiration, while during expiration the abdominal recti are seen to contract (Freund, Roos and Dodd, 1963), making abdominal surgery impossible at this stage. During deepening anaesthesia the muscles behave as if the spinal cord were becoming paralysed from below upwards. The recti no longer contract during expiration and the limb muscles relax. Ether anaesthesia is normally maintained at this level, the second plane of the third stage of Guedel's classification of the levels of anaesthesia (Guedel, 1937), both for superficial and for lower abdominal operations. Once it has been achieved, the concentration of anaesthetic can usually be reduced. On the other hand, if it is found that anaesthesia has lightened, as shown by a return of abdominal muscle tone, by an increase in respiratory rate or even by breath-holding, the concentration should be increased by 5 per cent. It may be necessary to assist breathing by working the bellows for a few breaths. Normal breathing will often return if the surgeon interrupts his work for a few seconds.

During ether anaesthesia the patient will be observed to take an extra deep breath every 2 to 3 minutes. This is a normal physiological event, believed to restore the surface tension-lowering effect of the surfactant lining of the alveoli. Figure 8.1 shows this happening in a young man breathing 5 per cent ether. The average tidal volume was about 400 ml but the deep breaths were nearly twice this. Deep breaths occur even in deep ether anaesthesia and should not be taken as a sign of lightening anaesthesia!

If anaesthesia is allowed to become deeper than recommended, the intercostal muscles and the peripheral part of the diaphragm, which is innervated by the intercostal nerves, will become paralysed. When this happens the central part alone is responsible for drawing air into the lungs. Its contraction becomes rather jerky, pulling the mediastinal structures, including the trachea, suddenly downwards with each breath. This is known as tracheal tug. When tracheal tug occurs, it will be noticed that the intercostal muscles are pulled inwards and the supraclavicular fossae

Fig. 8.1   Slow speed recording of respiratory volume during ether anaesthesia,
showing intermittent physiological deep breaths

Table 8.1 The signs of ether anaesthesia.

Stage	Respiration	Eyes	Voluntary muscles	Circulation
1 Analgesia	normal rhythm	voluntary control, pupils small	normal tone	normal rate, rhythm
2 Delirium	irregular, with coughing, breath holding and laryngospasm, phonation	lash reflex lost, pupils dilate but react to light, eyes 'roving'	spontaneous movement of limbs, tone may be increased, recti contract in expiration	frequency increases, ectopics
3 Surgical anaesthesia	regular with little expiratory pause and deep breaths every 2–3 minutes	no lid reflex, pupils central, small but dilating with increasing depth; pupils react to light	tone reduced with no limb movements, contraction of abdominal recti disappears	Heart rate rapid, pulse full, BP maintained
Deep anaesthesia	tracheal tug	light reaction disappears	intercostal paralysis	BP falls
4 Medullary paralysis	apnoea	fixed dilated pupils	flaccid	hypotension, bradycardia

drawn downwards during inspiration. Similar chest movements accompanied by tracheal tug are seen in upper airway obstruction and after giving sub-paralytic doses of muscle relaxants. This type of respiration is inefficient because the tidal volume is inevitably reduced and as a result, in spite of an increasing frequency of respiration, the oxygen saturation of the blood will tend to fall. The cause of the condition must be determined, because the treatment is different in each case. In this case, the concentration of ether should be reduced. The diaphragm pushes the abdominal contents downwards in the same jerky manner, making it very difficult for the surgeon to work within the abdomen. For this reason, although the abdominal muscles are flaccid, deep ether anaesthesia is not suitable for upper abdominal surgery. At the same time, it may be found that the degree of abdominal relaxation provided by the recommended level of surgical anaesthesia is inadequate. In such cases, other means of obtaining abdominal muscle relaxation must be employed.

Oxygenation during ether anaesthesia

Although the use of air is adequate in light surgical anaesthesia at the level recommended here, patients who may under-ventilate should be given additional oxygen at the rate of 2 litres per minute. This includes patients with chronic lung or heart disease, those with abdominal tumours which may interfere with respiration, and particularly patients undergoing Caesarian Section. Temporary apnoea should be treated by giving a few deep breaths with the bellows. However, the most important rule to follow when giving an ether anaesthetic is to avoid deep anaesthesia and not to go beyond the point at which the abdominal muscles are relaxed during expiration. Under normal circumstances a patient breathing ether/air will have an oxygen saturation above 90 per cent (Izekono et al., 1959), but if respiration is depressed, the saturation will fall. Cole and Parkhouse (1963) observed cyanosis during the maintenance period in 7.4 per cent of their patients which they were able to relieve either by adding oxygen or by assisting ventilation. Cyanosis was more common during operations in the Trendelenberg, lithotomy or lateral positions. Weitzner et al. (1959) have estimated that cyanosis will not be apparent until the oxygen saturation has fallen to 50 per cent. In any case cyanosis will not occur unless about 5 gm haemoglobin per 100 ml blood are in the reduced state, so it will not be seen in severely anaemic patients. Clearly then, cyanosis indicates a serious degree of hypoxaemia.

Further studies of oxygen and carbon dioxide tensions during ether/air anaesthesia were made by Markello and King (1964). They found that patients given 50–75 mg pethidine in their premedication suffered falls in arterial oxygen tension to a mean level of 71 mm Hg during halothane-assisted induction. On the other hand, in those given hyoscine alone the lowest level was 88 mm Hg, equivalent to 94 per cent saturation. Later on, after the halothane had been turned off and the operations had begun, the mean levels rose to 83 mm Hg (92 per cent saturation) and 91 mm Hg (95 per cent saturation) respectively. This information is shown in graphical form in Figure 8.2 in which the solid dots represent mean figures for patients given hyoscine alone, while the open circles represent those given pethidine in addition. 'Plane 1' values are those from the end of induction, which was assisted by 4 per cent halothane. 'Post stim' values are those

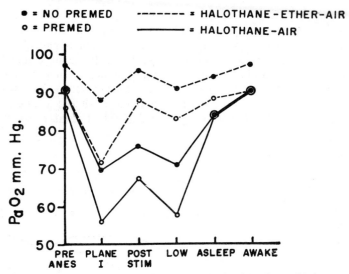

Fig. 8.2   Arterial oxygen tensions during anaesthesia with ether and halothane. See text for further explanation

immediately after the start of surgery, which normally stimulates respiration, while 'low' figures represent the lowest values during operation. Note that both the pre- and post-operative oxygen tensions were lower in those given pethidine, but that in both groups the mean level on waking was the same as before operation. Marshall and Grange (1966) observed very similar results in patients given 50 mg pethidine with atropine for premedication. These findings suggest an increased level of intra-pulmonary shunting during ether anaesthesia. It is interesting to note that in all cases the carbon dioxide tensions were at or below the normal level. Although hypoxia does not occur during a properly given ether/air anaesthetic, particularly if opioid premedication is avoided, it should be remembered that periods of apnoea, underventilation, coughing or breath-holding will be rapidly followed by a fall in oxygen tension (Cole and

Parkhouse, 1961). Arterial hypoxaemia (sub-oxygenation) will mean that vital tissues run the risk of permanent anoxic damage. The effect of oxygen starvation on the brain, whether due to hypoxaemia or to hypotension, will range from slightly delayed recovery from anaesthesia to a prolonged period of restlessness, followed sometimes by quite marked mental changes. The effect on the heart will be of progressive failure, accompanied by bradycardia or if sudden in onset, of cardiac arrest.

Circulatory effects of ether anaesthesia

Although cardiac output and arterial pressure are usually well maintained during spontaneous respiration with ether, it should be remembered that they depend on an active sympathetic nervous system. In patients who are under treatment with sympathetic blocking drugs (including certain sedatives and tranquillisers), in some apparently normal subjects and in elderly patients, this may not apply. In these patients it will be noted that an increase in the inspired concentration of ether will lead to a fall in arterial pressure and cardiac output (Gregory et al., 1971). For this reason the

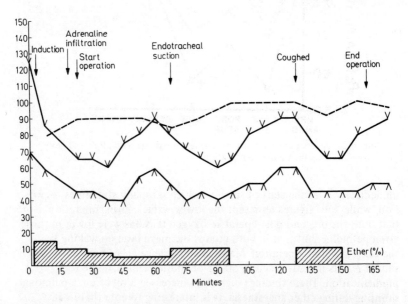

Fig. 8.3   Heart rate and arterial pressure during anaesthesia, showing a hypotensive response to ether. Heart rate (– beats per min.) and arterial pressure (∨∧ mm Hg) in a 35 year old woman having a partial thyroidectomy. Anaesthesia was induced with thiopentone 250 mg, followed by suxamethonium 40 mg to assist endotracheal intubation. Artificial respiration was given until the effect of the relaxant wore off. Note the well marked hypotensive response to 10 per cent ether

arterial pressure should be measured in every patient at regular intervals, and particularly when concentrations greater than 10 per cent are being used. Figure 8.3 is the record of a patient who showed a hypotensive response to ether. Dysrhythmias, usually in the form of ectopic beats, are quite common under ether anaesthesia and are probably an expression of increased sympathetic activity. No attempt should be made to treat them, either with local anaesthetics or with beta-adrenergic blockers, because an alarming fall of arterial pressure may follow. The occurrence of ectopic beats will be accompanied by a fall in cardiac output.

Patients undergoing abdominal operations will often be observed to have low arterial pressures during traction on the bowel, for example, during vagotomy (Farman, Gool and Scott, 1961). An example of this is shown in Figure 8.4. Possible reasons for this are reflex inhibition of the heart via the vagus, kinking of the inferior vena cava (which reduces venous return flow) or retraction of the gall-bladder during ether anaesthesia

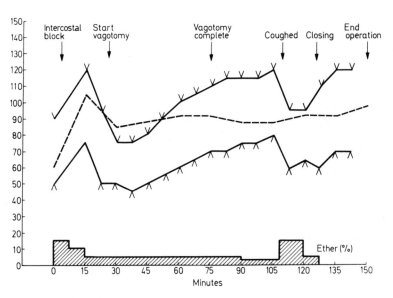

Fig. 8.4   Heart rate and arterial pressure during anaesthesia, showing hypotension during vagotomy. Heart rate (– beats per min.) and arterial pressure (v∧mm Hg) in a 26 year old man undergoing vagotomy and gastro-enterostomy. Anaesthesia was induced with 300 mg thiopentone and intubation assisted with 50 mg suxamethonium. Intercostal block was performed with 20 ml 2 per cent prilocaine with adrenaline, which probably accounts for the early peak of arterial pressure and heart rate. The arterial pressure fell at the start of the vagotomy but recovered spontaneously before it was completed. It fell again later when the ether concentration was increased to 15 per cent after the patient coughed.

(Vandam, Schweizer and Kubota, 1962). These responses occurred within a few seconds and were accompanied by a mean reduction of one third in cardiac output, slowing of the heart and a mean fall of 40 per cent in mean arterial pressure.

The use of other agents

Halothane has undoubted advantages as an induction agent but is less satisfactory for the maintenance of anaesthesia. It is a comparatively poor analgesic and the concentrations required in the absence of nitrous oxide depress both respiration and circulation. Bryce-Smith and O'Brien (1956) investigated its use when vaporised with air. They found that at least 2 per cent vapour was required. The frequency and volume of respiration both decreased, except when the stimulus of operation was present. Cyanosis, bradycardia and hypotension were common. They concluded that halothane is not a suitable agent for vaporisation with air alone. Oxygen supplementation is therefore needed throughout anaesthesia. Their experiences were confirmed by Markello and King (1964), whose findings are illustrated in Figure 8.2.

Trichloroethylene is also a useful induction agent. Unlike halothane it is a good analgesic but it causes rapid, shallow breathing and recovery may be prolonged. It is a poor muscle relaxant and is unsuitable as the sole agent when given in air. However, it has been used very successfully to provide analgesia, both on its own and in higher concentrations (0.5–1 per cent) to supplement relaxant anaesthesia (see below).

The combination of draw-over halothane and trichloroethylene has advantages. It is not practical to mix the two agents but if two O.M.V. vaporisers are available they can be placed in series. The halothane vaporiser must be placed upstream of the trichloroethylene vaporiser, otherwise trichloroethylene will condense in the halothane vaporiser. For superficial operations 1 per cent halothane is given with 0.5 per cent trichloroethylene. This avoids the respiratory and circulatory depression caused by higher concentrations of halothane. The trichloroethylene can be turned off some minutes before the end of the operation, as its analgesic effect is long-lasting. The great advantage of this technique is that it provides satisfactory anaesthesia within a few minutes of the start of induction, which may be with an intravenous agent or with the inhalational drugs only (Scott, Pilberg and Vellacott, 1971, Boulton, T. B., personal communication). The other advantage is that the mixture is not flammable.

The degree of abdominal relaxation provided by surgical anaesthesia with ether or the halothane-trichloroethylene combination will be sufficient for some operations on the lower abdomen, such as appendicectomy or repair of a strangulated inguinal hernia, in which it is not necessary to pack away much bowel. It will also be suitable for Caesarian Section in which profound relaxation is not needed for closure because by this time the abdominal wall is already lax. In other cases in which a wide exposure is required, or for operations on the upper abdomen, it will be necessary to employ some additional means of obtaining muscle relaxation. For the doctor working on his own it will usually be preferable to do an inter-costal block. On the other hand, if skilled assistance is available, a long-acting muscle relaxant, combined with artificial respiration, may be preferable.

The use of intercostal block for muscle relaxation in abdominal surgery (Farman, Gool and Scott, 1962)

With this technique, which is described in Chapter 11, abdominal relaxation is ensured by means of bilateral intercostal nerve block combined with light general anaesthesia of the type described above. Respiration remains un-impaired because a deep plane of anaesthesia is not attempted, so the doctor can safely entrust the patient to an assistant. The block is usually performed after the induction of general anaesthesia. This means that he can himself induce anaesthesia and perform endotracheal intubation before handing over to an assistant. The method is simple and quick, ten nerves being blocked in two or three minutes. It is best to perform the block before scrubbing up for the operation. There is always enough time for it to become effective before the operation begins.

The degree of relaxation produced by intercostal block is as great as that provided by the conventional relaxant techniques, but the success of the method depends in part on the moderate degree of muscle relaxation produced by ether. For this reason if one or two segments are not properly blocked, the relaxation of the abdomen is not noticeably impaired. If the operating time exceeds the duration of the block, it is possible to perform the block again. However, in most cases it will be sufficient to deepen anaesthesia slightly to assist closure of the abdomen.

Intercostal block leaves intact the autonomic innervation to the viscera and therefore does not interfere either with traction reflexes, depression of which may produce hypotension, or with other circulatory reflexes. A combination of light general anaesthesia with intercostal block does not depress circulation in the same way as spinal or epidural anaesthesia. The volume of ventilation is unaffected by the block (Farman, Gool and Scott, 1961) and oxygenation of the blood remains normal (Magbagbeola, J. A. O., personal communication).

The use of relaxants and artificial respiration   (Macintosh, 1955)

This technique can be used as an alternative to intercostal block for producing muscle relaxation for abdominal operations. The main advantage is that low concentrations of anaesthetics can be used to maintain uncon-sciousness, with correspondingly quicker recovery from anaesthesia. At the same time, particularly in elderly or poor risk patients, there is less risk of circulatory and respiratory depression. A technique which depends on artificial respiration is essential for operations within the chest in which the normal pattern of breathing is impossible, and advisable in operations in the face-down position. It is also indicated in very fat patients, those with large abdominal tumours, ascites, or when the lateral or Trendelenberg positions are used. For intra-cranial operations this technique is used to ensure efficient CO_2 elimination and to prevent vasodilatation, which occurs with high ether concentrations, and which is associated with raised intra-cranial pressure. It is not a technique which can be applied by unskilled anaesthetists because proficiency in artificial respiration, described in Chapter 5, is essential.

Anaesthesia is induced in the way described in the previous chapter, an endotracheal tube being passed. If suxamethonium has been used to assist intubation, the patient should be permitted to recover from this relaxant. Once spontaneous respiration has returned, a dose of long-acting relaxant should be injected intravenously. This will act within about one minute. Immediately respiration is depressed by the relaxant, artificial respiration is begun. It is essential that the lungs should be ventilated continuously during the period of action of the relaxant. The anaesthetic concentration is immediately reduced to a level sufficient to ensure a light level of unconsciousness and analgesia.

Experience suggests that equipotent doses of all anaesthetics are more or less equally toxic (Parkhouse and Simpson, 1959), and the actual choice of agent is not important. Nitrous oxide is commonly used in large hospitals, but other agents can equally well be used. Air is the carrier gas used with the E.M.O. system, enriched with oxygen when indicated. Ether, halothane, trichloroethylene or methoxyflurane can be employed, vaporised in the E.M.O. (in the case of ether) or in the O.M.V. Of these ether will be the only possible agent if the E.M.O. is the sole vaporiser, but trichloroethylene, halothane or methoxyflurane will be preferable if there is an explosion risk, as in thoracic surgery, when the surgeon wishes to use diathermy within the chest.

Effective concentrations for this purpose are: ether 3 per cent, halothane 0.5 per cent, trichloroethylene 0.5 per cent and methoxyflurane 0.3 per cent. If anaesthesia becomes too light, these concentrations may be doubled until the patient settles down. It is usually wise to try turning the anaesthetic agent off a few minutes before the end of the operation. Trichloroethylene has been reported to cause prolonged post-operative drowsiness (Parkhouse, Holmes and Tunstall, 1963). However Prior (1972) did not find the degree of drowsiness after operation was unacceptable. Indeed some degree of sedation may be an advantage, especially as the patients experience a worthwhile period of analgesia. Prior also observed that when trichloroethylene was used to supplement relaxant anaesthesia (as opposed to nitrous oxide or ether) the doses of relaxant needed to control respiration were greatly reduced, although the actual relaxation of the abdominal muscles wore off in the normal way, suggesting a central effect on respiratory control. Halothane is the least effective analgesic, but the other agents will provide considerable post-operative analgesia. On grounds of cost, safety and effectiveness, trichloroethylene is the agent of choice.

In the conditions under which this method is likely to be used, it is usually impossible to measure the volume of ventilation and the movement of the chest must therefore be watched extra carefully throughout. Vigorous ventilation is essential to prevent arterial hypoxaemia. A mechanical ventilator should be used where possible because it is more reliable than hand ventilation (De Castro, 1962) and it leaves the anaesthetist free to monitor the patient. If a Wright Respirometer is available, it can be attached to the outlet of the non-rebreathing valve. It is a considerable advantage to be able to do this because the size of each breath can be checked. Marshall and Grange (1966) showed that it is necessary to ventilate hard enough to lower the arterial carbon dioxide tension to below 25 mm Hg (normally 35–45 mm Hg) in order to maintain a normal oxygen tension when using ether/air. They found that a minute volume in the region of 19 litres, about two and a half times that needed to maintain a PCO_2 of 40 mm Hg is required. The reason for this is that the difference between the alveolar and arterial oxygen tensions $(A - a\ DO_2)$ increases markedly under these conditions, probably due to increased intra-pulmonary shunting. The cerebral vasoconstrictor effect of a low arterial PCO_2 will be counteracted by the cerebral vasodilatation caused by ether (Boyan, 1963).

Poppelbaum (1960) has employed relaxant ether/air anaesthesia, given with an E.M.O. inhaler, for thoracic operations. In patients with normal lungs oxygen saturations are maintained even when only one lung is being ventilated. When the lungs are affected by disease this often proves impossible and arterial saturations fall, sometimes rapidly.

Wakai (1963) found in healthy patients that the smallest minute volume needed to keep the oxygen saturation above 95 per cent was the same as the patient's resting minute volume before the induction of anaesthesia. By employing a facemask, non-rebreathing valve and Wright spirometer it is possible to measure this volume before the anaesthetic is begun. This appears to be the most practical guide to the level of ventilation required.

The choice of relaxant will depend on which drugs are available and on the condition of the patient. D-tubocurarine, which lowers arterial pressure, can be given in a dose of 30 mg when conservation of blood is essential in healthy patients. The use of gallamine (120 mg for an average adult) is associated with an increase in cardiac output which may cause rather heavy bleeding. However, this drug may be the relaxant of choice in elderly or shocked patients in whom its cardiac stimulating effect is valuable. For general purposes pancuronium bromide (dose 6 mg for an average adult) is the relaxant of choice. If at any time during the procedure the patient shows any reaction, additional relaxant is given. In the case of curare, 10 mg is a suitable dose, for gallamine 40 mg, and for pancuronium 2 mg.

When the end of the operation is in sight, no additional relaxant should be given. If relaxation is inadequate during closure, then the concentration of ether should be increased to 5 per cent and the volume of ventilation increased. When the skin is being closed the concentration should be cut to zero, but ventilation should continue as before. The action of the relaxant is reversed with atropine and neostigmine. It is usual to inject 1 mg of atropine intravenously as soon as skin closure is complete; this will produce a tachycardia. Once this has been established, neostigmine 2−3 mg is injected in increments of 1 mg. If more than 3 mg is given bradycardia may develop: this should be treated by giving a further 0.5 mg dose of atropine. Ventilation with air is continued until the patient shows signs of reacting to stimuli such as pinching the ear. As soon as he starts to react, oxygen (2 litres per min) is added to the inspired mixture. When he makes an attempt to breathe, the artificial respiration should be timed to coincide with these spontaneous efforts. Finally, assistance to respiration may be stopped and the patient permitted to breathe oxygen-enriched air. The endotracheal tube can then be removed, as described in Chapter 10.

Chapter Nine

The End of Anaesthesia

This chapter describes not only the actual ways of ending anaesthesia, but also the care of the patient in the immediate post-operative period. During recovery the patient is still under the influence of the anaesthetic drugs and is to a varying extent incapable of protecting himself from harm. The responsibility of the anaesthetist does not end until the patient has fully recovered from these effects.

The end of the operation

When the patient has been breathing spontaneously, with or without an intercostal block, the ether should be turned off some time before the operation actually finishes. The interval will depend largely upon the length of the operation. During an unexpectedly short procedure the patient may barely have reached a surgical level of anaesthesia before the operation is complete, and the ether will have to be turned off hurriedly. If this happens, usually due to miscalculating the likely duration of operation, the tissues will not be fully saturated and recovery will be fairly rapid. For short operations it will often be better to use halothane, either alone or in combination with trichloroethylene, for the sake of quick induction and recovery. Halothane should be kept at the maintenance concentration for the duration of the operation, but trichloroethylene should be turned off a few minutes before the end.

For longer operations, the concentration of ether will have been progressively reduced, to 3—5 per cent. Even with these concentrations the ether can safely be turned off 10—15 minutes from the end. For the majority of operations this means the beginning of closure of the wound and although this is one of the most painful parts of the operation, ether is such a powerful analgesic that the patient seldom moves. If it is necessary to resume anaesthesia, start with 5 per cent ether to avoid coughing, increasing the concentration to 10 per cent if necessary.

When the ether has been turned off, there is little point in making the patient continue to breathe through the apparatus, so the mask can be removed from the patient's face. A clear airway must still be maintained, as described in Chapter 5. When an endotracheal tube has been used, it should be left completely undisturbed until the operation is over because any attempt to remove it at this stage will make the patient cough. The vapour condenser should be left in place, but the valve and corrugated tubing can be removed.

Extubation

The endotracheal tube should only be removed when it is certain that the patient is breathing adequately and that it will be impossible for him to aspirate secretions or blood into the lungs. If there are secretions in the trachea a bubbling sound will immediately become apparent when the vapour condenser is removed. They should be aspirated in the tube with a soft sterile catheter until they can no longer be heard bubbling. Secretions, blood and the throat pack (if used) must be removed from the pharynx before extubation. This is best achieved by suction, although in an emergency mops may have to be used. A non-traumatic rigid pharyngeal suction end should be used (Argyle Type 1100 or Yankauer's with wide-bore olive tip). Electric powered suction is best although some foot-operated models (Cape or Ambu, Figure 4.24, page 66) are adequate. A laboratory-type filter pump attached to a water tap is a very efficient source of suction. The pharyngeal airway is removed and the laryngoscope gently introduced into the mouth, commonly revealing a pool of mucus lying in the pharynx, which should be aspirated. The suction end should then be used to clear the nasopharynx (by passing the tip behind the soft palate) and the lower part of the pharynx by temporarily lifting the tongue with the laryngoscope to allow access for the suction end. Lastly, secretions may be removed from the nose by applying the suction to one nostril while occluding the other; this is repeated on the other side. Suction catheters should only be passed into the nose with extreme care because bleeding frequently follows. Blind naso-pharyngeal suction with a catheter is far less effective than the method described above. The pharyngeal airway is then replaced.

Oxygen (4–6 litres per minute) should be added to the inspired mixture for 2–3 minutes before the tube is taken out, during the period of pharyngeal suction. This will ensure that there is a high concentration of oxygen in the lungs. It is most conveniently done by re-attaching the valve and tubing and adding oxygen via the E.M.O. If the patient then coughs or holds his breath when the tube is removed he will be protected (temporarily) against the risk of hypoxia. For the maximum safety the patient should be turned onto his side before the actual removal of the tube. The cuff is deflated (making sure that the pilot balloon has emptied) and the tube smoothly withdrawn. The facemask should then be attached to the valve and the administration of oxygen continued until the patient is again breathing quietly.

The reversal of long-acting relaxants has been described in Chapter 8. A few patients who have been artificially ventilated during operation may be incapable of breathing spontaneously afterwards. Examples are patients with gross metabolic acidosis or hypothermia, those who have chronic lung disease or have had lung resections, some patients with head injuries, some patients who have received intraperitoneal antibiotics (Emery, 1963) and those who have been overdosed with premedicant drugs or with ether (Cole and Parkhouse, 1963). In these cases artificial respiration must be continued and is best performed by a mechanical ventilator. If this is not available, hand ventilaton should be used employing relays of operators if necessary, until the patient is again capable of breathing spontaneously.

Position of the patient

The ideal position of the patient emerging from anaesthesia is lying on his side, for the following reasons:

1) The tongue falls to the side instead of backwards, allowing air passages to remain clear without the need for support to the jaw. The head must remain extended on the neck, however.

2) Secretions, blood and regurgitated stomach contents can run from the mouth and are less likely to be inhaled.

3) Pressure is removed from pressure areas on the patient's back; a change in posture will relieve strain on joints and ligaments. The position adopted is shown in Figure 9.1: the patient may have a small pillow under his head, but the level of the head should not be higher than the body. A larger pillow can be used to support the upper leg.

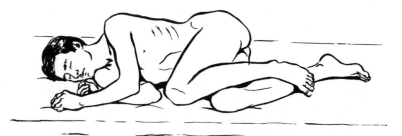

Fig. 9.1   Post-operative position of the patient. He is lying on his side with knees bent up to prevent him falling over. Pillows may be used to support the head and the upper leg

The patient should either be transferred directly from the table to his bed or placed on a special post-operative trolley. Direct transfer to the bed is ideal, but it is not always easy to bring the bed to the theatre, and some form of trolley is usually employed. The ideal post-operative trolley is

shown in Figure 9.2. It has vertically acting drop sides, a thick rubber
mattress and a cradle for an oxygen cylinder. It can be tilted so as to
lower the patient's head and raise his feet simply by pulling a lever and
pressing the end of the trolley downwards. This is a very important feature
because it means that any nurse can operate it in the event of a patient
vomiting or becoming hypotensive. The trolley should have a tray for the
patient's notes, mouth gag, mops, foot-operated sucker, etc.

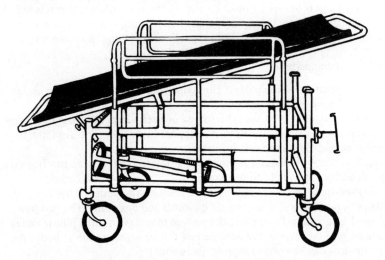

Fig. 9.2   Post-operative trolley (Made by A. C. Daniels). This trolley has a
head-end tilt control, sides which can be raised, a drip stand and provision
for an oxygen cylinder, resuscitation equipment and the patient's notes

The recovery room

It is both safe and economical to concentrate patients who have just had
operations and are recovering from their anaesthetics in a room near the
theatre. This idea is not new. In 1863, Florence Nightingale wrote 'It is
not uncommon, in small country hospitals, to have a recess or small room
leading from the operating theatre, in which patients remain until they
have recovered'. The advantages are that the patient does not have to
be moved while still in the unconscious state, the doctor is nearby if anything should go wrong and one nurse can care for more than one patient.
The recovery room should be equipped with electrically powered suction,
oxygen, a sphygmomanometer (preferably wall mounted), good lighting
and with some means of communicating with the theatre staff. If a number
of operations are to be performed on the same day, it will often be

worth designating one ward as the recovery room for that day, even if it is not possible to provide a purpose-built recovery room.

The patient will normally remain here until he has recovered consciousness and is stable, he can respond to simple commands, and it is considered safe to return him to the ward. This will usually occur within 20–30 minutes of the end of the operation (Leatherdale, 1966). It is important to have a good nurse in charge. Patients in a recovery room need not be segregated according to sex.

Complications in the post-operative period

1) *Hypotension*

It will be found that the commonest complications in the immediate post-operative period are circulatory. Hypotension may be associated with bradycardia or a low blood volume. Bradycardia is treated with atropine 0.25–0.5 mg intravenously. Low blood volume hypotension is usually associated with other signs of shock, namely vasoconstriction, tachycardia and cyanosis. Oxygen (4 litres per minute) should be given by a mask, such as the Harris mask, so as to raise the inspired concentration to about 50 per cent. The patient should be tilted by raising the foot of the trolley or bed by 5–10 degrees. Fluid replacement should be given urgently. Further treatment will depend on the cause of the hypovolaemia.

2) *Post-operative pain*

Patients who have been anaesthetised with ether benefit from its strong analgesic action during the first few hours after operation (Parkhouse, Lambrechts and Simpson, 1961). Trichloroethylene and methoxyflurane have a similar action, but analgesia is not appreciable after nitrous oxide or halothane anaesthesia. The worst pain is experienced by patients having upper abdominal operations. Lower abdominal operations, hernia repairs, head and neck, limb and superficial operations give rise to pain in a descending order of severity. All patients having major operations, especially abdominal operations or hernia repairs, should be prescribed an analgesic to be given after operation. Morphine 0.1–0.15 mg per kg, or pethidine 1–1.5 mg per kg are suitable. Both these drugs may cause respiratory or circulatory depression and may encourage vomiting (Dundee et al., 1965). Pentazocine 0.5–1 mg per kg has the advantage of having less emetic action and of being apparently non-addictive.

These drugs are described in Chapter 3. It should be emphasised that the safest way to give analgesics is 'little and often'. Large doses at infrequent intervals cause respiratory and circulatory depression and vomiting, followed by periods in which the patient experiences agonising pain. A time interval of 2–3 hours is about right. When prescribing analgesics it is therefore better to specify a moderate dose, to be given when needed, than large doses at fixed 'safe' intervals. Severely ill patients should be given small doses intravenously (morphine 1–2 mg, pethidine 10–20 mg, pentazocine 10–20 mg). Such doses can be repeated after 5 minutes if analgesia is not achieved, without the risk of overdosage. The intravenous route should always be used in patients suffering from shock.

3) *Post-operative vomiting*

It is widely believed that ether is responsible for severe and prolonged vomiting during recovery from anaesthesia. Careful enquiry among patients who have received ether does not support this belief (Holmes, 1965) and in fact ether is little different from other anaesthetics in this respect. Indeed, when controlled respiration with a relaxant is used, ether is superior to other agents. Post-operative vomiting is commoner in females and will be encouraged by the use of morphine-like drugs for premedication and post-operative analgesia. Psychological, cultural and racial factors appear to be important. In Britain about one third of patients vomit after receiving ether via the E.M.O.

Post-operative vomiting usually occurs after recovery of consciousness. The danger of aspiration of vomitus is reduced if the patient is nursed in the lateral position. Repeated vomiting can be treated by the use of an anti-emetic drug, such as perphenazine (5 mg IM for an adult, 0.1 mg per kg).

Chapter Ten

Anaesthesia in Children

It is essential when anaesthetising children to bear in mind certain anatomical and physiological differences from adults. These assume the greatest importance in the smallest children. Anaesthesia and surgery in children, especially in infants, carry a high risk. The simplest and safest possible methods should always be used, combined with an understanding of these special factors.

Anatomy and physiology

Infants

These are taken as children aged less than one year, while neonates are infants of less than one month. Development in the first few months of life will depend to some extent on the maturity of the child at birth. At first the child is incapable of doing much more than eating and sleeping, almost all the metabolic activity being concerned with breathing, the function of the heart and with body growth. There is little reserve capacity in any physiological system.

The lungs are small in relation to body size. At birth the child is able to withstand the anoxia associated with apnoea of several minutes duration, but this will lead to the development of metabolic acidosis. Breathing may be irregular, with periods of apnoea associated with hypoxia or prematurity. The frequency of respiration is normally between 30 and 40 breaths a minute. The tidal volume depends on the body weight and is about 5 ml per kg per breath. The normal minute volume for a 2.5 kg infant is about 0.5 litres, which accords well with the rate of metabolism. The functional residual capacity is small and is further limited in the supine position by the pressure of the abdominal contents, particularly if the abdomen is distended. In order to increase the minute volume, the infant increases the frequency of respiration, which it can do with comparatively little extra effort.

The heart in the neonate is relatively immune to hypoxic damage. The rate is rapid, around 100 at rest, rising to nearly 200 beats a minute on crying or struggling. Hypoxia causes bradycardia which is reversed rapidly when the cause is corrected. The normal haemoglobin level at birth is around 18 grams per 100 ml but this falls to about 12.5 grams per 100 ml by the age of three months. The haemoglobin is mainly of the foetal type, which carries more oxygen at low tensions than the adult type. The proportion of foetal haemoglobin falls during the first few weeks. Anaemia may occur during the neonatal period due to haemorrhage or malaria (Mansell, M. E., personal communication).

The metabolic rate is higher at birth than in the adult. The oxygen consumption is about 6 ml per kg per minute, rising to a peak at 6 to 8 months and then falling gradually off towards the adult level of 4 ml per kg per minute. Hypoglycaemia, which may cause brain damage, is common in post-mature neonates, with levels below 16 mg per 100 ml. Neonates, especially when premature, have little ability to regulate their temperature, and readily become hypothermic. This tendency is exacerbated by illness, cold surroundings, exposure and anaesthesia which causes vasodilatation and increased heat loss. The fall of temperature under anaesthesia is greater when controlled respiration with relaxants is used, and when cold blood is transfused. Hypothermia is every bit as common in the tropics as in temperate climates, especially in air-conditioned buildings (Farman, 1962) and is associated with difficulty in breathing and failure to feed. Conversely, dehydration can cause a rise in temperature. Infants, especially when newborn, should be brought to the theatre well wrapped up, in an incubator if necessary, and should be exposed for the minimum length of time. If possible the air-conditioning should be turned off. The infant should be placed on a heated pad if artificial respiration is to be used or if the operation is likely to be prolonged, and should be wrapped in insulating material wherever possible. The temperature should be recorded both during the operation and immediately it is over. If it is below 35°C (95°F), active warming should be given immediately.

The prothrombin level falls over the first few days of life and then rises again. The resulting prolongation of clotting time may be associated with haemorrhage. Physiological jaundice is common in the first few weeks of life, probably because the immature liver is unable to conjugate bilirubin. Other enzyme systems may be immature and drugs either given to the mother before the birth of the baby or given directly to the baby, may produce unexpected effects.

The anatomical configuration of the upper airways in infants differs from that in older children and adults. The tongue is large and the epiglottis is curved instead of flat. The larynx is higher in the neck and the vocal cords slant upwards and backwards. The narrowest point is not at the glottis but at the cricoid ring, a point to be remembered when passing an endotracheal tube. The cough reflex is relatively immature at this age.

Older children

Metabolic rate declines gradually throughout childhood but the rate of
fall becomes less over the age of about eight. The resting heart rate becomes
lower with increasing age. Systolic arterial pressure is 85–90 mm Hg in
infants, rising to about 100 mm Hg at the age of ten (Smith, 1968).
It should be remembered that once the deciduous teeth begin to come out,
there will always be the possibility of loose teeth in this age group. Nasal
obstruction due to enlarged adenoids or secretions is not uncommon.
Apart from these factors the older child differs little from the adult.

Anaesthesia

Infants

Infants are premedicated with atropine alone; 0.25–0.3 mg of aqueous
solution may be given orally one hour before operation. Alternatively, half
of this quantity can be given by intramuscular injection a quarter of
an hour beforehand. Monitoring of vital signs by adult methods is usually
impossible in small children. It is therefore best to rely on the precordial
stethoscope. This should be of the diaphragm type and is strapped to the
chest so that it can pick up both respiration and heart sounds. It is best to
lead the sound to one ear only, leaving the other free. A monaural stethoscope of this type can be improvised from drip tubing and a brachial
stethoscope diaphragm (Boulton, 1966).

Maintenance of a clear airway in infants is not the same as in older
children. The antero-posterior diameter of the head is large and the head
tends to flex when the baby is lying on a flat surface. It is useful to place
a folded towel transversely beneath the neck and shoulders to extend the
atlanto-occipital joint and to stabilise the head. Extension of the head and
support of the chin may actually cause respiratory obstruction. Lifting
the jaw by pressing beneath the angle of the mandible is usually effective,
but it is to some extent a matter of trial and error. When consciousness
is lost, it may be helpful to insert the appropriate size of lubricated oral
airway. If this appears to make the obstruction worse, the airway should
immediately be withdrawn.

Open-drop ether

For minor operations the open-drop method can be employed. Only ether
should be used, as other agents have an unpredictable effect and may lead
to respiratory and circulatory depression. Oxygen 0.5 litre per minute
should be led under the mask with a fine catheter. The infant's face is
covered with gamgee tissue in which a hole has been made for the nose
and mouth. An infant wire-frame mask with 12 layers of gauze is placed

on top of the gamgee and an airtight fit obtained. Ether is allowed to drop on to the mask at a steady rate. Patience is required and the rate of dropping should not be so fast that the gamgee becomes soaked with ether or the patient coughs or holds his breath. The ether should be dropped over the whole area of the mask, not just at one point. The rate may be increased slightly once the nose and air passages become insensitive. The anaesthetist should listen for every breath and immediately correct any obstruction. If coughing or breath-holding occurs, ether should be withheld until respiration is again regular. The signs of anaesthesia with ether are the same as in adults and have been described in Chapter 8. An additional sign in babies is relaxation of the hand grip under surgical anaesthesia.

Using the E.M.O. as a constant-flow vaporiser

The deadspace of the non-rebreathing valves and connections used for larger children and adults are too great for infants and children below the age of 3 or 4. Use of the adult apparatus will lead to exhausting hyperventilation and asphyxia. Moreover, the inspiratory flowrates generated by such children are too small for satisfactory vaporisation of ether in the E.M.O. For these reasons the techniques described for adults are not suitable. The paediatric entrainer was designed to provide a flow of oxygen-

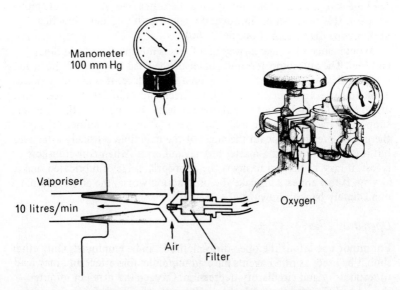

Fig. 10.1   The Paediatric entrainer. The oxygen flow is regulated until the manometer reads 100 mm Hg, when the total flow will be 10 litres per minute

enriched air through the E.M.O. in order to vaporise the ether (Farman, 1965, 1966). It consists of a fine jet, through which oxygen passes into a Venturi-shaped tube. Air is drawn in and mixes with the oxygen. The entrainer is plugged into the air inlet of the E.M.O. (Figure 10.1).

Alternative means of providing a flow may be used. Nitrous oxide and oxygen may be used (5.0 litres per minute of oxygen and 5.0 litres per minute of nitrous oxide) delivered from a gas anaesthetic machine, via the E.M.O. flowmeter attachment or with the Entonox premixed nitrous oxide/oxygen apparatus of Latham (Latham and Parbrook, 1967). The use of the Revell circulator, an oxygen driven pump, has also been reported (Sodipo, J. O., personal communication). Whichever source of gas flow is used, the E.M.O. is used as a constant-flow or plenum vaporiser. However, it was designed to give the indicated concentration with the intermittent flows encountered during spontaneous respiration. In order to deliver the correct concentration a total gas flow of about 10 litres per minute is needed (Epstein, H. G., personal communication). The concentration delivered at various gas flows and vaporiser settings is given in Table 10.1.

Table 10.1. Concentration (vol per cent) of ether delivered by the E.M.O. vaporiser at 26°C with constant gas flows (Figures supplied by Dr. H. G. Epstein).

		Dial setting (per cent)					
		2	3	4	6	10	15
Gas flows (l/min)	7	1.2	1.7	2.3	3.2	6.1	11.9
	9	1.5	2.7	3.5	5.4	9.9	13.8
	11	1.8	3.0	4.2	6.1	9.0	13.7

The paediatric entrainer is driven from an oxygen cylinder, preferably via a regulator (reducing valve), although even a fine control tap on its own will work. The actual flow of oxygen need not be measured. Instead, the pressure of the driving gas is measured with a clinical blood pressure manometer, which is attached to the side arm. This way of estimating flow depends on the fact that the rate of flow of gas through a fixed resistance varies with the driving pressure. The flow of gas from the cylinder is increased until the manometer reads 100 mm Hg, when the entrainer will deliver the correct flow of 10 litres per minute. Occasional adjustment of the control tap is needed during the course of an anaesthetic. A fine filter is provided to prevent dust entering the high pressure part of the entrainer and clogging the jet. If the jet were to become clogged the flow of driving gas would be less than indicated, with a corresponding reduction in the total flow provided. The jet can be unscrewed for cleaning if this should prove necessary. A wire gauze filter protects the air entry ports.

By using oxygen as the driving gas, an inspired oxygen content of about 35 per cent is achieved. Although this is clinically advantageous, overcoming most of the effects of ventilation-perfusion inequalities it renders an ether mixture explosive. When compressed air is used as the driving gas, the ether remains flammable but is no longer detonable (Macintosh, Mushin and Epstein, 1963). Patients lightly anaesthetised with ether tend to hyperventilate even when intubated, but for infants it is nevertheless safer to employ an oxygen-rich mixture to minimise the risk of hypoxaemia developing as a result of the patient coughing or holding his breath. If the use of diathermy or open flames is essential, a non-explosive agent must be used instead of ether.

The consumption of driving gas is 2 litres per minute, so that even in situations where oxygen supplies are low the running cost is not prohibitive. The entrainment ratio is 1.5:1. If the outflow from the entrainer is occluded the high pressure gas escapes through the air inlet holes and the maximum internal pressure achieved is 15 cm H_2O. This means that if the gases are prevented from escaping from the breathing circuit for any reason, the pressure in the apparatus will not rise above 15 cm H_2O which is unlikely to harm the patient. When in use the entrainer makes a low hiss, which becomes louder if the outlet is obstructed. The device has the advantages of low cost, economy, safety and simplicity. Although it was designed with the E.M.O. in mind, it can equally well be used with the O.M.V. to vaporise halothane or other agents.

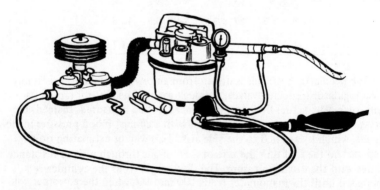

Fig. 10.2   The E.M.O. O.I.B., entrainer and Ayres' T-piece ready for use. Note that the magnet is *not* used on the bellows.

The entrainer is inserted into the air inlet of the E.M.O. The bellows and O.M.V. or B.S.I.U. are left in the circuit but the bellows is pushed down into the 'closed' position. The anaesthetic mixture is led to the patient via the delivery tube to a T-piece, one end of which leads to the

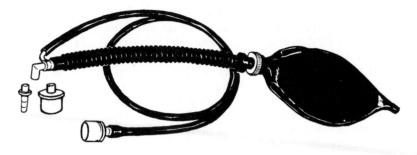

Fig. 10.3   Ayre's T-piece (Cambridge modification). The fresh gas delivery tube is bent back for the sake of neatness, while the patient end is bent down to fit either a facemask (via an adaptor) or an Oxford endotracheal tube connection

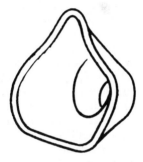

Fig. 10.4   The Rendell-Baker facemask

patient via a facemask or endotracheal tube (Figures 10.2 and 10.3). The facemask designed by Rendell-Baker (Figure 10.4) is by far the best. The other end has a reservoir tube, which should have a volume greater than the patient's tidal volume. Too short a tube will permit the baby to breathe room air. It is usual to employ a 25 cm corrugated rubber tube, 1 cm in diameter, for this purpose. Rees (1960) has modified this basic design by putting a 500 ml open-ended bag on the end of the reservoir tube which can be used for artificial respiration. The delivery tube of the Ayre's circuit is attached to the outlet of the O.I.B. in place of the long corrugated tubing. When the Penlon Bellows is used, the O.M.V. or B.S.I.U. remains on the downstream side of the bellows. The delivery tube is then attached to the outlet of the accessory vaporiser.

Harrison (1964) has measured the minute volumes of anaesthetised children. He found that in a one-year old child it will be 1.5 litres, in a three-year old child 2 litres, and in a five-year old 3 litres. He recommended that a fresh gas flow of 2.5–3 times the minute volume should be used with Ayre's T-piece to prevent rebreathing of expired air. The flow delivered by the entrainer is therefore adequate for the largest child likely to be anaesthetised by this method. The possible disadvantage of using a flow greater than three times the minute volume is that the resistance to expiration will be increased. Although a flow of 10 litres a minute may be unnecessarily high for neonates, the advantage of knowing the concentration of ether outweighs this disadvantage. From Harrison's figures it would seem that the peak expiratory flow in a child under one year will be less than 6.6 litres a minute. The maximum flow in the expiratory limb of the T-piece will therefore be 16.6 litres a minute (Peak expiratory flow plus a fresh gas flow of 10 litres a minute), so with a T-piece of 10 mm diameter as recommended by Ayre (1956), the resistance is likely to be negligible.

Anaesthesia with ether is induced by turning on the entrainer and setting the control dial to 4–5 per cent. The mask is lowered gently over the baby's face. The concentration is increased evenly until 20 per cent is reached. Because at this setting the concentration will still be rather less than indicated, it may be necessary to maintain it for longer than expected. Reliance should be placed on the signs of anaesthesia, rather than on the duration of exposure to a particular concentration. Care must be taken to ensure that the level of anaesthesia does not become too deep. If the B.S.I.U. is used, it should be charged only with trichloroethylene. In order to avoid wastage the entrainer should be turned on immediately before the start of induction. When using the O.M.V. with halothane to assist induction, it should be set to deliver 0.5 per cent only. The ether is then introduced in the usual way and the halothane turned off as soon as surgical anaesthesia is reached. For short procedures halothane can be used as the sole anaesthetic agent; 1–2 per cent vapour will be needed. The signs of anaesthesia are the same as for ether; the most important sign is muscular relaxation.

Endotracheal intubation

For certain operations endotracheal intubation is essential. The indications are similar to those in adults and are discussed in Chapter 5.

The common types of tubes and connections used in neonates are shown in Figure 10.5. The Cole neonatal type has a thick non-kinking wall for most of its length, while the tip, which passes the glottis, is much thinner. The Oxford tube has a built-in bend. Magill tubes in these sizes are likely to kink and are therefore less suitable than the other types. The best connections for this size of tube are the Oxford type. A straight infant-size

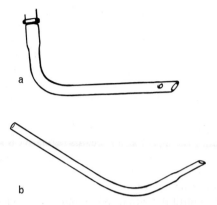

Fig. 10.5a   Oxford endotracheal tube with Oxford connector
    b   Coles pre-sterilised plastic tube (Made by William Warne)

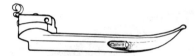

Fig. 10.6   Seward laryngoscope blade

laryngoscope blade is best. The Seward, Robertshaw, Oxford Infant and Anderson types are all suitable. The Seward is shown in Figure 10.6.

Before passing the tube, make sure that the laryngoscope is working. All connections should be ready; test that they fit each other correctly. The estimated size of tube, as well as one a size smaller than expected should be ready and lubricated with water-miscible jelly. The tube should never be a tight fit in the cricoid ring: the correct size is 0.5 mm smaller and will permit a small leak when the bag is squeezed. The approximate size is given in Table 10.2. Tubes of the Magill and Cole types with a continuous curve are supplied too long and have to be cut to size. The Oxford tubes, already of the correct length, do not need trimming.

Neonates are best intubated while awake. The child is wrapped in a towel to immobilise its arms and the assistant holds its head. Oxygen is first given

Table 10.2. Approximate sizes and lengths of endotracheal tubes needed in children of different weights

Weight (kg)	2	3	4	8–10	15–20
Diameter (mm)	2.5	3.0	3.5	5.0	6.0
Length (cm)	8	10	12	15	17

via a mask. The T-piece, mask and paediatric entrainer can be used if the air inlet holes are temporarily blocked off. The laryngoscope is then taken in the left hand and the lips parted by the fingers of the right hand. The blade is introduced and passed gently behind the tongue and lifted to expose the glottis. This should not prevent the child breathing if care is taken. The assistant then presses the larynx gently backwards and the tube is passed. Coughing is uncommon, but the child's breathing will often become irregular or stop altogether, so it is essential to connect the anaesthetic circuit immediately. Artificial respiration (see below) should be given for a few breaths until the infant again breaths regularly. Both lungs are auscultated with a stethoscope to ensure that the tube has not passed into one bronchus. The tube should then be fixed in place with strapping (see Figure 10.7). The ether concentration is then turned up to 10–15 per cent for a few minutes until the infant settles and ceases to move its limbs.

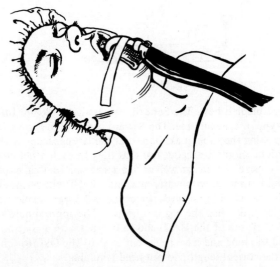

Fig. 10.7   Endotracheal tube and Ayre's T-piece fixed in place. The wide upper tube is the exhaust limb and the lower the fresh gas delivery tube

When surgical anaesthesia is reached as shown by relaxation of the hand grip, the concentration can be reduced to about 5 per cent.

For operations in the prone position or on the chest, when breathing would otherwise be inadequate or impossible, artificial respiration is continued throughout. In this case the concentration of ether should be reduced immediately to 5 per cent, otherwise dangerously deep anaesthesia will develop. The hand grip is relaxed when the depth of anaesthesia is suitable for the operation to begin. Beware of using a higher concentration than the minimum needed to maintain anaesthesia; between 3 and 5 per cent is usually enough.

Artificial respiration is performed by intermittently occluding the exhaust limb of the T-piece with the thumb, as shown in Figure 10.8. The flow through the E.M.O. and breathing circuit (derived from the entrainer) is 10 litres per minute, about 170 ml per second. When the outlet is occluded the whole of this flow is directed into the patient's lungs, just over 40 ml will enter the lungs in 0.25 seconds. An adequate minute volume will be achieved in the neonate by giving about 15 such breaths per minute. For older infants a longer period of occlusion will lead to a correspondingly larger tidal volume. The minute volume of a neonate is about 0.5 litres, rising to about 1.5 litres in a one year old child. In practice is is impossible to measure these volumes and reliance must be placed on watching the

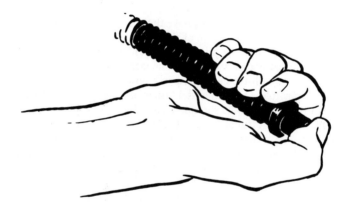

Fig. 10.8   Artificial respiration in an infant. The end of the exhaust limb of the T-piece is occluded intermittently

movement of the chest and controlling the tidal volume in the light of its expansion.

Before removing an endotracheal tube at the end of anaesthetic, the pharynx should be examined with the laryngoscope. Exposure of the glottis is not necessary. All secretions should be gently sucked out through a catheter. An oral airway is then inserted, not only for the patient to breathe through, but to prevent him biting and occluding the tube as he wakes up. The patient is then put on his side. The T-piece should remain attached during this manoeuvre so that the patient can continue to breathe the oxygen-rich mixture. The endotracheal tube can then be gently removed and the facemask substituted. The patient may hold his breath or cough so he should be allowed to breathe the oxygen-rich mixture until respiration is again regular.

Children aged 1–4 years

Premedication

Because of their high metabolic rate, children need rather large doses of premedicants (on a body weight basis) than adults. Oral premedication is given 2 hours before the operation is due. Atropine 0.02 mg per kg and diazepam 0.5–1 mg per kg usually ensure a calm, well prepared patient. In excitable children or those in whom a quiet post-operative period is essential (such as certain plastic operations, neurosurgery and tonsillectomy), droperidol 0.25 mg per kg may safely be given in addition. Chloral or other tranquillisers may be used, but opioids and barbiturates should not be given because they depress respiration.

Children in this age group do not have the special anatomical features described in neonates. Maintenance of the airway is more like that in an adult, with head extension the primary requirement, although support of the jaw and use of an oral airway may be needed. However, it is best to begin the induction with the child lying in a position of comfort, disturbing him as little as possible. Once unconsciousness is achieved, it is best to support both the head and the shoulders on a thin (5 cm) pillow.

When endotracheal intubation is not required, the open-drop method may be used. To make induction quicker and pleasanter 3 ml of halothane or trichloroethylene may be dropped onto the mask slowly from a glass or nylon syringe (disposable plastic syringes may dissolve in these agents). Ether is then introduced at a fairly rapid rate, distributed evenly over the mask. As the ether evaporates it cools and eventually frost will form on the mask due to the condensation and freezing of exhaled water vapour. The mask should then be changed for a fresh one. The rate of dropping of ether is reduced once surgical anaesthesia is achieved.

As an alternative the E.M.O. may be used as a constant flow vaporiser in conjunction with Ayre's T-piece. The paediatric entrainer or a similar source of flow will be used, as already described. Trichloroethylene rather than halothane should be used in the B.S.I.U. Halothane may be given via the O.M.V., but the concentration should never exceed 1 per cent when ether is to follow. The ether is introduced steadily in increments of 1 per cent every four breaths, up to 20 per cent in healthy children, 15 per cent in ill children. The halothane must be turned off as soon as surgical anaesthesia is reached, otherwise the patient will become too deeply anaesthetised.

Halothane alone may be given with the O.M.V. for short procedures or when there is a risk of explosion due to the use of diathermy. In this case up to 3 per cent vapour will be needed for induction and 1.5–2 per cent for maintenance of anaesthesia. When nitrous oxide (65 per cent oxygen) is used as the carrier gas, these halothane concentrations may be reduced by 0.5 per cent because of the anaesthetic and analgesic effect of the gas.

Ketamine is useful for short superficial operations in children. Its great advantage is that it is rapid in onset but its duration of action is long enough for the majority of minor procedures. As in adults it can also be used for the induction of anaesthesia, which can then be continued with an inhalational agent (see Chapter 7). The intravenous dose is about 2 mg/kg, which acts within a few seconds and lasts about five minutes. Muscle tone and arterial, intracranial and intra-ocular pressures are increased. Nystagmus makes ketamine unsuitable for most ophthalmic procedures, while muscle rigidity prevents the performance of abdominal operations. However, ketamine has proved valuable for children who are distressed by the prospect of operation and who will not accept inhalational or intravenous drugs. Terrifying dreams during emergence appear to be very uncommon in children (Boulton, 1971).

Endotracheal intubation

Children too big for awake intubation should be intubated while breathing spontaneously under general anaesthesia. There is no need for relaxants in children this size. The patient is anaesthetised with ether as described above until surgical anaesthesia is achieved. The advantages of intubating under ether are that the signs of anaesthesia are clear cut (eyes central, pupils slightly dilated, abdominal muscles relaxed), respiration is stimulated and anaesthesia does not become light too rapidly. No attempt must be made to pass the tube until anaesthesia is deep enough. Local analgesia with lignocaine (10–20 mg) is useful if there is no risk of aspiration of blood or secretions. A metered aerosol which delivers 10 mg per puff is particularly useful here because the dose can be ry easily be controlled. The maximum safe dose of lignocaine is 3 mg per kg and this must not be exceeded.

The lengths and sizes of tube are given in Table 10.2. The types of tube have been discussed already (page 151). The infant laryngoscope blades can be used in this age group.

Intubation may be performed under halothane alone, but again sufficient depth of anaesthesia must first be achieved. Respiration is depressed by halothane and the patient may appear deeply anaesthetised during light anaesthesia, only to cough violently when an attempt is made to intubate. Anaesthesia lightens rapidly when the agent is withdrawn, so intubation must be performed without delay. It is necessary to use up to 3 per cent halothane until the abdominal muscles relax and the pupils are moderately dilated. The laryngoscope is then inserted and the glottis sprayed with 10 or 20 mg lignocaine when permitted. No attempt is made to intubate at this stage. The chances are that this alone will have made the patient cough. The facemask is reapplied and the halothane administered for a few minutes more until the local anaesthetic has made the larynx insensitive. The laryngoscope is re-inserted and the glottis expose; the tube should then pass with ease.

Artificial respiration

In larger children the limited maximum inspiratory flow rate of about 170 ml per second means that the duration of inspiration will be prolonged to one second or more if reliance is placed on occlusion of the T-piece. For these children the Rees open-ended bag is preferable (Rees, 1960). However, when such a bag is squeezed there is the danger that some gas will return up the delivery tubing. Not only would this hinder inflation of the lungs, but the gases would make three passages through the ether vaporising chamber instead of only one, resulting in a dangerously high concentration of vapour. To prevent this, the bellows unit is always placed between the vaporiser and the breathing circuit, solely for the sake of its non-return valves, with the bellows itself immobilised (Farman, 1965; Austin, 1970). With this method the limits of pressure and flow set by the entrainer can be exceeded. The lungs are inflated by temporarily occluding the outlet of the bag between the thumb and forefinger, while at the same time squeezing the bag with the other fingers of the hand, as shown in Figure 10.9. At the end of the breath, the air is allowed to escape from the bag.

It is possible to employ an endotracheal tube in a child without the use of a flow source such as the entrainer. A right-angle suction type of endotracheal connector, such as the Cobb, must be fitted to the tube. Anaesthesia

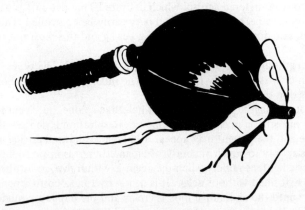

Fig. 10.9   Artificial respiration in a larger child. The open-ended bag is squeezed while the outlet is temporarily occluded

is induced by the open-drop method and the tube passed in the usual way. Artificial respiration is given by compressing the bellows at the same time that the suction hole is occluded with the finger of the other hand (Cole and McClelland, 1961). A non-rebreathing valve is not used with this method. The disadvantages are that both the anaesthetist's hands are occupied and that the arrangement is not suitable for spontaneous breathing in these small children. The Aga Polyvalve, which has a low deadspace (1.34 ml) and the Ambu valve are suitable for this age group. A special paediatric bellows of small diameter has been developed. A normal excursion of this bellows blows a smaller volume of air into the lungs than in the case of the adult bellows. The adult bellows can be used, provided the tidal volume is strictly limited. Artificial respiration may also be given with Ayre's T-piece by attaching the patient outlet of the non-rebreathing valve to the exhaust limb (Bethune, D. W. personal communication). The fresh-gas inlet of the T-piece is left open. When the bellows or bag is compressed sufficient flow is produced to inflate an infant's lungs, in spite of the leakage of air from the fresh-gas inlet.

Older children

Children over the age of 3 or 4 can easily be anaesthetised using the methods described for adults. Appropriate reduction of dosage (on a body weight basis), of intravenous agents and relaxants must be made. However, a child can safely be anaesthetised with the same concentrations of ether as used for adults, but it must be remembered that induction of anaesthesia is much quicker. When inducing anaesthesia the kindest way is to work the bellows so as to blow halothane or trichloroethylene over the child's face until unconsciousness occurs, rather than attempting to get a good mask fit from the beginning (Sugden, 1970). Stetson (1966) recommends assisting each breath with the bellows during induction. It usually takes between 5 and 10 minutes to reach surgical anaesthesia. Great care must therefore be taken to ensure that the child is not exposed to the higher concentrations for more than the necessary time, otherwise anaesthesia will become too deep. At all times reliance should be placed on the signs of anaesthesia. As in adults, ill children should not receive more than 15 per cent ether.

Leatherdale (1966) describes the use of the E.M.O. inhaler in conjunction with the Boyle-Davis gag for adeno-tonsillectomy in children. The gag has a tube for insufflating the anaesthetic mixture into the pharynx. The delivery tubing of the Ayre's circuit is used to lead the mixture from the vaporiser to the gag. Anaesthesia is induced in the usual way, with the patient breathing spontaneously. When surgical anaesthesia has been reached, the surgeon inserts the gag into the patient's mouth while the anaesthetist changes the tubing. Any of the flow sources described above may be used, or the bellows and non-rebreathing valve employed as a pump. As this is a relatively wasteful method, it will be found necessary to use 8–10 per cent ether vapour for maintenance.

Chapter Eleven

Regional Anaesthesia

Drugs

It is best to become thoroughly familiar with one or two agents. Lignocaine has succeeded procaine as the most commonly used drug because of its greater potency and safety combined with quicker onset and longer duration of action (1–1½ hours). 0.5 per cent is used for infiltration and sensory nerve blocks and 1 per cent for motor nerve blocks. Bupivicaine in half the above strengths is used when prolonged analgesia is required. Drugs used for spinal anaesthesia are discussed later, while all these drugs are described in Chapter 3.

Toxic reactions to local anaesthetics are most commonly due either to intravascular injection or to gross overdosage. The danger is minimised by infiltrating only while the needle is being advanced or withdrawn and, in the case of nerve blocks, by making an aspiration test. Maximum safe doses are given in Chapter 3. The toxicity of any given dose of drug is less when a dilute solution is used than with a stronger solution because low concentrations are less rapidly absorbed into the bloodstream. Absorption is also delayed by adding adrenaline to a strength of 1:200 000 (0.1 ml of 1:1000 adrenaline in 20 ml of local anaesthetic), which will not only reduce the toxicity but will prolong the duration of analgesia. Adrenaline containing solutions should be used for all blocks except those in organs with 'end arteries' (e.g. hand, fingers, toes, penis) in which there is a danger of gangrene. For infiltration and field blocks the spread of the local anaesthetic is helped by dissolving one ampoule of hyaluronidase at the time of mixing with adrenaline. Provided adrenaline is present, hyaluronidase does not increase the rate of absorption of the local anaesthetic.

The toxic effects of local anaesthetics are drowsiness, twitching, and respiratory depression, leading to convulsions and hypotension. These effects are due to the drug entering the bloodstream and their severity and rapidity of onset will vary with the concentration of the drug in the blood. Prompt treatment is essential; the patient should be given oxygen and assisted or artificial ventilation may be needed. Convulsions can be controlled rapidly by an intramuscular injection of 40—50 mg suxamethonium with hyalase; an endotracheal tube must be passed and artificial ventilation continued, assisted if necessary by further doses of suxamethonium. In convulsions, death is due mainly to anoxia and if this is prevented the patient will survive. Equipment for providing this treatment should always be at hand when nerve blocks are performed.

Equipment

If disposable equipment is not available, a pack should be made up containing 20 ml and 2 ml syringes with plain Luer hubs (locking hubs are not worth the trouble), gauze mops and 1.5 cm, 2.5 cm, 5 cm, and 10 cm needles. The needles are threaded into a gauze mop and the syringes rolled up in mops; everything is then rolled in a towel and tied with ribbon gauze. Two or three such sets should be prepared and autoclaved. They are opened on a tray or table top and the towel serves to keep it sterile. An assistant opens the ampoule of local anaesthetic, being careful not to contaminate the edge of the bottle, and pours the contents into a sterile mixing pot. He then opens an ampoule of adrenaline 1:1000 and the doctor draws up 0.1 ml for every 20 ml of solution, using the 2 ml syringe and adds that to the contents of the pot.

Equipment for spinal anaesthesia is described later.

Preparation of the patient

For small operations little preparation is needed. In the case of field blocks multiple injections may be distressing and it is both kinder and easier for the surgeon to sedate the patient well. Papaveretum 20 mg is suitable for the average adult, given an hour beforehand, but in excitable patients the dose may be increased or droperidol 5—10 mg added. If further analgesia is needed at the time of operation pethidine 25—50 mg or pentazocine 30—60 mg may be given slowly by intravenous injection. The patient should have voided beforehand and preferably not have eaten recently in case a general anaesthetic is needed or vomiting or a toxic reaction occurs.

The site of the block and the operation site (if different) should first be washed with soap and water after which the skin is prepared as for surgery. A gallipot and sponge holders are needed and the sterile mops from the pack used. The skin preparation solution should be allowed to dry before any injection is made.

Local infiltration

This is used for cutaneous and subcutaneous surgery, e.g. removal of a lipoma, gland biopsy, episiotomy, suture of wounds. 20 ml of 0.5 per cent lignocaine with adrenaline is drawn up and skin weals are raised at points around the operation site, using the 1.5 cm needle. A 5 cm needle is then attached and inserted through a skin weal. Lignocaine is injected while the needle is advanced just under the skin, first to one side and then to the other side of the operation site. The syringe is recharged and reinserted through another skin weal and the injection continued until the skin surrounding the operation site and the area beneath it has been infiltrated. The object is to raise a barrier of local anaesthetic solution all around the operation area. Injections must always be made with the needle on the move to avoid depositing a large quantity of solution in a blood vessel.

Nerve blocks

a)   *Pudendal block*
This is suitable for outlet forceps delivery and most breech deliveries. The pudendal nerve supplying the perineum is blocked in the region of the ischial spine. 50 ml of 0.5 per cent lignocaine with adrenaline is needed. A weal is first raised in the perineal skin between the fourchette and the anus. A 10 cm needle is then introduced first one one side and then on the other, alongside the lateral wall of the vagina. The needle is guided by a finger placed in the vagina until the tip reaches the ischial spin. 10 ml is injected to block the nerve as it leaves the pelvis and enters the perineum below the spine. A further 10 ml is injected into the labium on each side and another 10 ml beneath the skin and vaginal mucosa on the side chosen for the episiotomy.

b)   *Intercostal block*
This block is described mainly because of its use as an adjunct to ether anaesthesia, as mentioned in Chapter 8. Intercostal block with bupivicaine is also valuable in the treatment of chest injuries and for some operations on the chest and abdominal walls. The nerves are blocked posterior to the origins of the lateral cutaneous branches. This may be done by injecting in the posterior axillary line or at the angles of the ribs in the case of the upper segments. An assistant should stand on the other side of the supine patient with one hand beneath the shoulder and the other beneath the patient's hips, and should then pull the patient towards him, as shown in Figure 11.1. The upper arm should be allowed to fall forward to pull the scapula off the angles of the ribs. This gives a good exposure for all the nerves, including the twelfth nerve.

    The extent of the block is determined by the probable site of operation. Five segments are usually blocked on each side, except in robust patients in whom six segments are blocked, in all cases bilaterally. It is important to block both sides because one of the functions of muscle relaxation is to permit the retraction and packing away of abdominal contents from the field of operation.

    Lignocaine 1 per cent with adrenaline is the drug of choice when

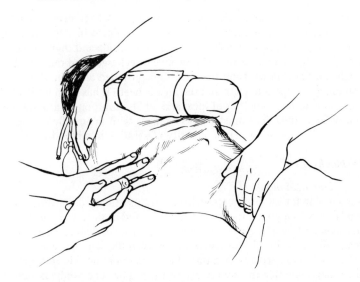

Fig. 11.1   Performing an intercostal block. The patient's arm is folded
across his chest in order to swing the scapula forward off the angles of the
ribs. An assistant pulls the patient over so as to expose the posterior ends of
the ribs

anaesthesia is maintained with ether, 2 ml being injected in the region of
each nerve, using a total of 200 mg of lignocaine (20 ml of 1 per cent
solution). If the operation time is expected to exceed about two hours,
20 ml of 0.25 per cent bupivacaine should be used. This will act for up
to nine hours (Moore et al., 1970) and will give useful-post-operative
analgesia. Solutions containing adrenaline should not be used when
patients are receiving halothane, trichloroethylene or chloroform because
of the risk of serious cardiac dysrhythmias.

The skin is cleaned and while the rib is palpated with the free hand a
2.5 cm needle is passed through the skin in a slightly cephalad direction so
as to strike the rib above the nerve to be blocked. The needle is gently
manoeuvred downwards until it can be advanced just beneath the lower
border of the rib. It is then pushed in a further 3 millimetres. As the
needle passes through the intercostal muscles there is a distinct feeling
of resistance which helps to locate the tip. 2 ml of solution is then injected,
as shown in Figure 11.2. If a swelling appears beneath the skin at the
injection site, the needle is too superficial and should be advanced further
so that it lies beneath the intercostal muscles. It is important that a syringe
is always attached to the needle throughout, to reduce the risk of a
pneumothorax if the pleura is pierced. A rare but dangerous complication

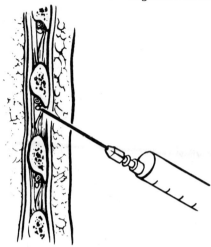

Fig. 11.2   Section of the chest wall, showing the ribs, intercostal muscles and the neurovascular bundle. Local anaesthetic solution is being injected

is the production of a bilateral pneumothorax. Care must be taken not to push the needle too far for fear of lacerating the lung, liver or spleen.

c)   *Axillary Block of the Brachial Plexus*
This block is ideal for operations on the hand and forearm. Pneumothorax and accidental block of the phrenic, recurrent laryngeal and vagus nerves or the stellate ganglion are impossible, so there is no contra-indication to bilateral block. The brachial plexus passes beneath the clavicle and into the axilla, accompanied by the axillary artery and vein. These vessels and the three nerves are enveloped in a well-defined sheath of connective tissue. Only the musculocutaneous nerve, supplying the lateral aspect of the upper arm, leaves the plexus above the level of the axilla and is not easily blocked by this route. This may present a problem if a tourniquet is to be used.

The patient lies with his arm abducted to a right angle and his forearm flexed and externally rotated. A soft rubber tourniquet is placed as high as possible round the arm to limit downward spread of the solution. The skin is cleaned and the axillary artery palpated. If it is not palpable the block will have to be abandoned. A needle 5 cm long is inserted into the neuro-vascular bundle as high in the axilla as possible, so that its tip lies just above the artery (figure 11.3). A distinct loss of resistance may be felt as the needle enters the bundle. The commonest mistake is to push the needle in too far, so that the tip lies deep to the bundle. If it is in the correct position it will move in time with the pulsation of the axillary artery. Paraesthesiae may be elicited by the needle, although it is not necessary to seek them.

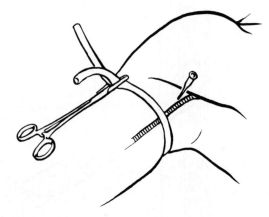

Fig. 11.3   Axillary block of the brachial plexus. The needle has been inserted into the neurovascular bundle alongside the axillary artery. The tourniquet prevents downward spread of the local anaesthetic solution

40—50 ml is needed for a complete block of the plexus, including the musculocutaneous nerve, depending on the size of the patient. 0.5 per cent lignocaine or 0.25 per cent bupivicaine may be used, depending on the duration of block desired. In either case the solution must contain adrenaline (1:200 000 or so) to limit the rate of absorption of this large volume of solution. 2—3 ml is left in the syringe, to be injected subcutaneously as the needle is withdrawn, to block the intercosto-brachial nerve supplying the medial aspect of the upper arm (Winnie and Collins, 1964).

d)   Ring block of finger or toe
This is used when one finger or toe is involved. 1 per cent lignocaine is used, without adrenaline (which will cause gangrene in these circumstances). With a 1.5 cm needle, 4 ml of solution is slowly injected on either side of the base of the digit, blocking the digital nerves. A rubber catheter is then drawn tightly round the digit and clipped with a haemostat. This not only prevents bleeding but stops the local anaesthetic being washed away.

e)   Field block for inguinal hernia repair
This block is used in patients who are unsuitable for spinal anaesthesia. For recurrent, sliding femoral and irreducible hernias extra infiltration may be needed during operation to stop pain caused by manipulation of the peritoneum. Gentle handling of the tissue is important and even in uncomplicated cases adequate premedication is essential. Obese patients cannot be given this block because of the dangerously large doses of local anaesthetic needed. 100 ml of 0.5 per cent lignocaine with adrenaline and hyaluronidase are used even in an adult of average build.

    With the patient lying on his side the 11th and 12th thoracic nerves are

each blocked with 2.5 ml of solution as they run beneath their ribs.
[See (b) — Intercostal block.] A weal is then raised one finger's breadth
medial to the anterior superior iliac spine. A 5 cm needle is passed
perpendicularly through this weal until it is felt to pierce the external
oblique aponeurosis. 20 ml of solution is deposited as the needle is
advanced, blocking the ilioinguinal and ilio-hypogastric nerves. A 10 cm
needle is then introduced over the anterior superior iliac spine and advanced
first sub-cutaneously and then intradermally, in the direction of the
scrotum, 1 cm below the inguinal ligament. 20 ml of solution is injected
during this stage.

The femoral nerve is blocked by passing the 5 cm needle through the
anaesthetised skin lateral to the femoral artery which is guarded by fingers
of the operator's free hand. The needle enters perpendicularly and 5 ml
of solution is injected as it is advanced. The needle is withdrawn and
re-directed, pointing laterally, and advanced again using another 5 ml of
solution. This is repeated a third time to give a fan shaped area of block.
A weal is raised over the pubic spine and the 5 cm needle is then used to
deposit 20 ml of solution along the pubic ramus, alongside the spermatic
cord, behind the pubis and into the attachment of the rectus abdominis.
Subcutaneous and intradermal injections are made along the line of the
skin incision, using a 10 cm needle introduced via the weal over the
pubic spine. 10 ml of solution is needed for this.

The remaining 10 ml is saved until later on during the operation when
the spermatic sympathetic plexus at the external ring and the peritoneum
and the genito-femoral nerve at the internal ring are infiltrated under
direct vision.

f)   *Field block for Caesarian section*
This is the safest anaesthetic for this operation and there is much to be
said from the point of view of both mother and baby for using it routinely.
80—100 ml of 0.5 per cent lignocaine with adrenaline and hyaluronidase is
needed. Opioids must not be used for premedication for fear of depressing
the baby, but may be injected intravenously after delivery. A tranquilliser
such as diazepam (5 mg intramuscularly) may be given beforehand.

With the patient lying first on one side and then on the other the 9th,
10th, 11th and 12th thoracic nerves are each blocked with 2.5 ml of
solution as they run beneath their ribs, using a 2.5 cm needle. Next a skin
weal is raised over the upper border of the symphysis pubis. A 5 cm needle
is then used to infiltrate behind the pubis, along both pubic rami and the
insertion of the abdominal rectus muscles using 20 ml of solution. A skin
weal is raised in the midline below the umbilicus (for a vertical skin
incision). With the 10 cm needle, 20 ml of solution is used to infiltrate
subcutaneously and intradermally along the line of the skin incision. The
remaining solution is kept until the abdomen has been opened. The

peritoneum between the uterus and the bladder is infiltrated with the solution. In addition to providing anaesthesia this is an aid to dissection.

g)   *Field block for the breast*
This can be used for breast abscesses and biopsies. 80 ml of 0.5 per cent lignocaine with adrenaline is needed. The patient should lie with her arm extended. The 3rd, 4th, 5th and 6th intercostal nerves are blocked in the axilla, using 2.5 ml of solution for each. A skin weal is raised at the lateral border of pectoralis major and the skin and subcutaneous tissue overlying this muscle infiltrated with the 10 cm needle. The line of infiltration extends to the sterno-clavicular joint and the needle must be reinserted halfway along this line. 40 ml of solution is used for this part of the block.

Intravenous local anaesthesia

This involves injecting local anaesthetic into a limb to which an arterial tourniquet is applied and is useful for operations on the hand, forearm and foot. 1 per cent lignocaine without adrenaline is used (adrenaline will cause gangrene of the limb).

A sphygmomanometer cuff is applied above the operation site and the systolic pressure measured. A self-sealing needle is then inserted into a convenient vein and secured with strapping (see Figure 7.1). The limb is then elevated for five minutes to drain off any surplus blood and the cuff inflated to about 30 mm Hg above the systolic pressure. The lignocaine is then injected into the vein through the needle. Anaesthesia develops in five to ten minutes. The volume of solution used depends on the size of the part to be anaesthetised. 15—20 ml are needed for a hand and 20—30 ml for a forearm or foot. The cuff must be kept inflated to prevent blood entering the limb and diluting the local anaesthetic. If the cuff becomes painful a second cuff must be applied distally and blown up before the first cuff is removed. The patient must be observed closely for 5 minutes after the cuff is finally removed in case a toxic reaction occurs due to the sudden release of local anaesthetic into the circulation.

Spinal anaesthesia

Principles
This method is suitable for operations on the lower abdominal, inguinal and perineal regions. It produces complete analgesia with profound muscular relaxation, quiet respiration and a small, contracted bowel. However it is contraindicated in shocked patients (the result of haemorrhage, toxaemia or dehydration), very anaemic patients, patients with severe heart disease, patients with very large abdominal tumours (which interfere with venous return to the heart), some patients with skin diseases affecting the lumbar

region, spinal deformities and diseases of the spinal cord, and children.

Local anaesthetic is introduced into the cerebrospinal fluid surrounding the cauda equina at lumbar puncture, blocking the spinal nerves in the subarachnoid space. As the spinal cord ends at the level of the first lumbar vertebra (except in children) it cannot be damaged by the needle. The sympathetic outflow extends from the upper thoracic to the second lumbar segment. Blocking the sympathetic fibres leads to vasodilatation and other signs of sympathetic paralysis. If this extends upwards for more than a few segments (beyond about T_{10}) a marked fall of blood pressure will occur. A block extending above this level is a 'high' spinal and is not recommended for the occasional anaesthetist. A 'medium' spinal block covers the segments from T_{10} or so to L_4 and is suitable for herniorraphy, lower abdominal operations and operations on the legs. A 'low' spinal (also called Saddle Block) affects only the sacral segments and is used for operations on the perineal region.

In the technique described here a small volume of hyperbaric ('heavy'), solution of local anaesthetic is injected into the subarachnoid space. This type of solution has a higher specific gravity than CSF and therefore passes downwards, its movement being determined by gravity and by the inclination of the spine. Thus if the patient is sitting up, the heavy solution sinks to the lowest part of the thecal sac, affecting the sacral roots only. If he lies on his back the heavy solution will not travel further than the lowest part of the thoracic curve and any unabsorbed drug will remain at this point.

Method

The drugs recommended here are procaine and cinchocaine. The former lasts for about an hour and the latter two to three hours. Procaine is available in ampoules containing 100 mg of crystals which are dissolved in 2 ml of CSF, cinchocaine ('Nupercaine') is presented in an ampoule containing 3 ml of hyperbaric solution in a strength of 1:200 (0.5 per cent) in 6 per cent glucose. Both these solutions are used in the same way and the choice depends on the duration of operation and the quality of the aftercare available for those patients whose operations end before their blocks wear off. Adrenaline is not used.

A 2 ml syringe, 1.5 cm needle, an introducing needle (Sise type) and a very fine lumbar puncture needle with a stylet (10 cm 22 S.W.G.) and a short bevel (45 degrees) are required. The ampoule of spinal anaesthetic and an ampoule file are wrapped in gauze mops with the syringes and needles and two towels, and the whole lot packed up in another towel and autoclaved. Procaine crystals and cinchocaine solution can be autoclaved two or three times if not used, (see Chapter 3).

The patient should be bathed and shaved and well sedated, as described at the beginning of the chapter. A stethoscope and sphygmomanometer cuff are fitted on the arm and a self-sealing needle inserted into a vein and secured with strapping. For a low spinal block, the patient sits on the operating table with his feet on a stool, and with knees flexed, leaning forward, hands clasping his ankles. For a medium spinal he lies on his side on the table with a pillow under his head and a rolled-up towel under his loin to prevent sagging of his spine. The table is tilted a little, head up for a woman and head down for a man, to make the spine level. The patient flexes his body and rests his head against his knees so as to enlarge the intervals between the lumbar spinous processes.

Wearing a mask the doctor should scrub up and don gloves. The sterile pack is laid on a table or tray and the outer towel unfolded, exposing the contents. The skin is cleaned and two towels laid diagonally across the patient, leaving a triangular area over the lumbar spine uncovered. 0.5 ml of cinchocaine solution (or 0.5 per cent lignocaine in the case of a procaine block) is drawn up. A line connecting the iliac crests crosses over or just above the fourth space which is located by palpating one crest through the towel. The injection is made into the third or fourth lumbar interspace. A skin weal is raised in the midline over the chosen space and the subcutaneous tissue beneath it infiltrated. The introducing needle is then inserted in the midline between two spines. It points slightly towards the patient's head and is advanced into the interspinous ligament, as shown in Figure 11.4. At this stage the doctor should sit down or kneel on the floor and steady the introducing needle with a hand resting against the patient's back. The

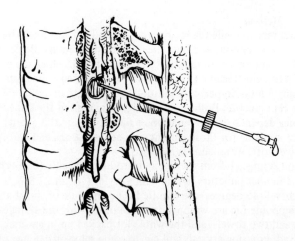

Fig. 11.4   Sectional diagram of the lumbar spine. A Sise introducer has been passed into an interspinous ligament. The spinal needle has been directed via the ligamentum flavum, extradural space and dura mater into the subarachnoid space in the region of the cauda equina

introducing needle is used to aim the spinal needle which is passed through it and advanced. If correctly placed it will pierce the ligamentum flavum with a distinct feeling of resistance. If bone is struck the needle is withdrawn and the direction of aim of the introducing needle checked. The needle may not be quite in the midline, it may be pointing too high or too low or the patient's back may not be sufficiently flexed. The needle is advanced again until the tip passes the ligamentum flavum. Before any change of direction it must be withdrawn into the introducing needle. If necessary another interspace should be tried. Use of an introducing needle simplifies the use of a fine, flexible spinal needle, which should never need to be bent as it is merely advanced into the subarachnoid space. The introducing needle also protects the spinal needle from contamination by skin organisms or the skin preparation solution, both of which can give rise to inflammation within the subarachnoid space. The shaft of the spinal needle should likewise never be handled.

Once through the ligamentum flavum the stylet is removed and needle advanced very gently through the dura, which may be felt as a slight loss of resistance. The bevel should be placed so as to divide rather than cut the longitudinal fibres of the dura. At this point CSF should flow out of the needle. If not, rotate the needle through 180 degrees, reinsert and remove the stylet (holding the hub firmly with the other hand) and try advancing or withdrawing the needle very gently. If necessary get the patient to strain so as to raise the CSF pressure. If after all this no CSF flows another space must be tried or a general anaesthetic given. When clear CSF is obtained reinsert the stylet.

Draw up the cinchocaine and again holding the hub firmly take out the stylet and attach the syringe. Withdraw a little CSF to confirm that the tip is correctly placed, and inject the cinchocaine steadily. In the case of procaine attach the empty syringe, withdraw 2 ml of CSF and reinsert the stylet. Empty the CSF into the ampoule of procaine crystals and agitate until they are dissolved. Re-attach the syringe and make the injection steadily. After the injection withdraw the syringe, spinal needle and introducing needle together and cover the puncture site with a dressing.

For a low spinal the dose is 1 ml (50 mg in the case of procaine). The injection is made with the patient sitting as described above, after which he should remain in position for 4–5 minutes until the local anaesthetic is 'fixed'. He should then lie down with his head and shoulders raised on a pillow. For a medium block the injection is made with the patient lying on his side. For a unilateral block the dose is 1.5 ml (75 mg procaine). The patient should lie on the side of the operation, where he should remain for 4–5 minutes until the solution is 'fixed'. For a bilateral block (for an inguinal or lower abdominal operation) the dose is 2 ml. The patient is turned onto his back immediately the injection is made and the table tilted 15 degrees head downwards until the anaesthetic is 'fixed'. A steep Trendelenberg (head down) position should not be adopted for at least 10—15 minutes after the injection lest the heavy solution should pass upwards to the diaphragm.

Complications

The period immediately after the injection is critical. The blood pressure should be checked every minute for the first fifteen minutes. This is best done by an assistant who also measures the level of sensory analgesia every minute with a swab soaked in ether. He should call out his findings to the doctor who will by now be scrubbing for the operation. The blood pressure may fall as the block develops. The assistant should continue to call out the blood pressure every five minutes during the remainder of the operation. He will reassure the patient and carry out any further treatment ordered by the doctor. If the patient's colour remains good and he is comfortable a fall in pressure will need no treatment, but if the systolic blood pressure falls below 60 mm Hg or pallor, cyanosis, sweating or retching develop, a vasopressor should be given. A small dose is injected intravenously and a large dose intramuscularly to produce an immediate and sustained effect. In addition oxygen should be given and the head-down tilt retained until the vasopressor has acted. Hypotension due to sub-arachnoid block is usually accompanied by bradycardia. Sudden hypotension occurring later in the operation may be due to blood loss (accompanied by tachycardia) or to traction on abdominal organs or the peritoneum.

Respiratory depression may be due to hypotension, in which case the respiratory centre becomes hypoxic and respiration is usually gasping in character. Breathing will improve when the hypotension is cured. The other cause is overdosage with local anaesthetic, leading to a high block involving the intercostal and even the phrenic nerves. In this case respiration may become jerky due to tracheal tug and then become progressively shallower. A block of this extent will certainly be accompanied by hypotension. Treatment therefore consists of giving a vasopressor drug, followed immediately by artificial respiration if the breathing does not return. Nausea may result from hypotension or from bowel traction. In the latter case it will be improved by the slow intravenous injection of an opioid.

Post-operative care

After the operation the patient should be lifted very gently because sudden bumping may precipitate hypotension. He should be nursed with a slight head-down tilt until the block has worn off. Remember that his legs and lower trunk will remain analgesic and will need to be positioned carefully. The blood pressure should be taken every ten minutes until all sensation has returned.

Post-operative complications can be troublesome. Urinary retention may occur in the first day or so and should be treated by neostigmine 1 mg subcutaneously every four hours, although catheterisation may also be needed. Pain at the injection site is usually transient and responds to physiotherapy. Headache occurs in about 10 per cent of cases and may last for a week. It is attributed mainly to leakage of CSF from the site of dural puncture and the incidence is lessened by the use of a fine needle for the puncture, avoiding coughing and straining afterwards and by keeping the patient flat on his back for 24 hours. Analgesics may be needed. Meningism may follow contamination of the CSF with red cells, particularly after a traumatic puncture. Lumbar puncture should be performed at another interspace and the CSF examined for cells and organisms. Septic meningitis due to a non-sterile technique should be treated with large doses of antibiotics if permanent neurological damage is to be avoided. However, major neurological sequelae are extremely rare if a proper technique is followed.

References and Bibliography

Adams, A. K. and Barnett, K. C. (1966) Anaesthesia and intra-ocular pressure. *Anaesthesia* **21**, 202.

Austin, T. R. (1970) Use of a Farman entrainer and EMO vaporiser with I.P.P.V. *Brit. J. Anaesth.* **42**, 363.

Ayre, P. (1956) The T-piece technique. *Brit. J. Anaesth.* **28**, 520. (Refers to Ayre, P. (1937) *Lancet* **1**, 561.)

Badoe, E. A. (1968) Pulmonary and cutaneous fluid loss in the Ghanaian. *W. Afr. Med. J.* **17**, 236.

Baraka, A. and Gabali, F. (1968) Correlation between tubocurarine requirements and plasma protein pattern. *Brit. J. Anaesth.* **40**, 89.

Batten, R. L. (1961) *The Surgery of Trauma in the Tropics.* London, Edward Arnold.

Baxter, C. R. and Shires, G. T. in Shires, G. T. (Ed). *Care of the Trauma Patient.* McGraw-Hill, London, 1966.

Beecher, H. K., Francis, L. and Afinsen, C. B. (1950) Metabolic effects of anaesthesia in man: acid-base balance during ether anaesthesia. *J. Pharmacol. exp. Ther.* **98**, 38.

Benke, A. (1959) The EMO Apparatus. A new portable apparatus for anaesthesia and resuscitation. *Wien med. Wschr.* **109**, 803.

Bhalla, S. K., Rama Rao, K. R., Subramaniam, C. S. V. and Rao, L. N. (1967) Chloroform — A study of over 500 cases. *Indian J. Anaesth.* **15**, 88.

Bhardwaj, V. B. and Coghlan, C. J. (1965) A simple vaporiser for halothane for use with the EMO ether inhaler. *E. Afr. Med. J.* **42**, 344.

Boulton, T. B. (1971) Editorial. *Anaesthesia* **26**, 125.

Boulton, T. B. (1966) Anaesthesia in difficult situations: (3) General anaesthesia. *Anaesthesia* **21**, 513.

Boulton, T. B. and Cole, P. V. (1966a) Anaesthesia in difficult situations: (1) What would I do if . . .? *Anaesthesia* **21**, 268.

Boulton, T. B. and Cole, P. V. (1966b) Anaesthesia in difficult situations: (2) General anaesthesia — general considerations. *Anaesthesia* **21**, 379.

Boulton, T. B. and Cole, P. V. (1968a) Anaesthesia in difficult situations: (7) Routine preparation and pre-operative medication. *Anaesthesia* **23**, 220.

Boulton, T. B. and Cole, P. V. (1968b) Anaesthesia in difficult situations: (8) Special Preparation — Blood, Fluids, electrolytes and drugs. *Anaesthesia* **23**, 385.

Boyan, P. (1963) General anaesthesia with minimal equipment. *N.Y. State J. Med.* **63**, 829.

Bryce-Smith, R. (1964) Halothane Induction Unit. *Anaesthesia* **19**, 393.

Bryce-Smith, R. and O'Brien, H. D. (1956) Fluothane: A non-explosive volatile anaesthetic agent. *Brit. Med. J.* **2**, 969.

Burton, A. C. (1965) *Physiology and Biophysics of the Circulation.* Year Book Medical Publishers, Chicago.

Clementsen, H. H. (1963) EMO inhaler and the Ambu bag. *Brit. Med. J.* **2**, 1409.

Cole, P. V. and McClelland, R. M. A. (1961) Use of the EMO inhaler and Oxford Inflating Bellows. *Mission Med. Bull.* **12**.

Cole, P. V. and Parkhouse, J. (1961) Blood oxygen saturation during anaesthesia with volatile agents vaporised in room air. *Brit. J. Anaesth.* **33**, 265.

Cole, P. V. and Parkhouse J. (1963) Clinical experience with the EMO inhaler. *Postgrad. Med. J.* **39**, 476.

Collis, J. M. (1967) Three simple ventilators. *Anaesthesia* **22**, 598.

Crul, J. F., Kelan, M. and Linssen, G. H. (1967) Untitled paper delivered at symposium on DehydroBenzperidol — Fentanyl, Moscow, May 23—24.

Cullen, D. J., Eger, E. I., Stevens, W. C., Smith, N. T., Cromwell, T. H., Cullen, B. F., Gregory, G. A., Bahlmann, S. H., Dolan, W. M., Stoelting, R. K. and Fourcade, H. E. (1972) Clinical signs of anaesthesia. *Anesthesiol.* **36**, 21.

Dardel, O. V., Holmdahl, M. H. and Norlander, O. P. (1966) A new modular system for anaesthesia and resuscitation (The Aga Polyvalve and the Aga Anestor Militor). *Acta Anaesth. Scand.* Suppl. 26.

Das Gupta, D. and Deval, D. B. (1970) EMO Vaporiser: Expiratory valve. *Brit. J. Anaesth.* **42**, 808.

De Castro, B. Jr. (1962) The EMO vaporiser using the technique demonstrated by Sir Robert Macintosh. *Proceedings 1st Asian and Australasian Congress of Anaesthesiology.*

Dripps, R. D. and Severinghaus, J. W. (1955) General anaesthesia and respiration. *Physiol. Rev.* **35**, 741.

Dundee, J. W. (1956) *Thiopentone and other thiobarbiturates.* Livingstone, Edinburgh.

Dundee, J. W., Kirwan, M. J. and Clarke, R. S. J. (1965) Anaesthesia and premedication as factors in post-operative vomiting. *Acta. Anaesth. Scand.* **9**, 223.

Emery, E. R. J. (1963) Neuromuscular blocking properties of antibiotics as a cause of post-operative apnoea. *Anaesthesia* **18**, 57.

Epstein, H. G. and Macintosh, R. R. (1956) An anaesthetic inhaler with automatic thermo-compensation. *Anaesthesia* **11**, 83.

Epstein, H. G. (1958) Principles of inhalers for volatile anaesthetics. *Brit. Med. Bull.* **14**, 18.

Etsten, B. E. and Li, T. H. (1960) Effects of anesthesia upon the heart. *Amer. J. Cardiol.* **6**, 706.

Farman, J. V. (1971) Apparatus for general anaesthesia in the small hospital. *Tropical Doctor* **1**, 29.

Farman, J. V. (1968) "Diplomas and Specialization". *Middle East J. Anaesth.* **1**, 620.

Farman, J. V. (1965) Economical anaesthesia overseas: air-entrainment device for use with draw-over vaporisers in children. *Brit. Med. J.* **2**, 1428.

Farman, J. V. (1962a) Heat losses in infants undergoing surgery in air-conditioned theatres. *Brit. J. Anaesth.* **34**, 543.

Farman, J. V. (1962b) The problem of anaesthesia in the underdeveloped countries. *Brit. J. Anaesth.* **34**, 897.

Farman, J. V. (1966) The use of an air-entrainment device in conjunction with a draw-over vaporiser. A method for small children. *Proc. 2nd. Europ. Congr. Anaesthesiol.* 486. (*Acta. Anaesth. Scand., Suppl.* **23**).

Farman, J. V. (1961) The use of the EMO apparatus for ether anaesthesia in the smaller hospital. *W. Afr. Med. J.* **10**, 355.

Farman, J. V., Gool, R. Y. and Scott, D. B. (1962) Intercostal block in abdominal surgery — a method for the single handed surgeon. *Lancet* **1**, 879.

Farman, J. V. and Powell, D. (1969) The performance of disposable venous needles and cannulae. *Brit. J. Hosp. Med. Suppl.* 37.

Francis-Lau, L. (1964) General anaesthesia with the EMO apparatus using air. *W. Indian Med. J.* **13**, 12.

Freund, F., Roos, A. and Dodd, R. B. (1963) Expiratory activity of the abdominal muscles in man during general anaesthesia. *J. Appl. Physiol.* **19**, 693.

Fullerton, W. T. and Turner, A. G. Exchange transfusion in treatment of severe anaemia of pregnancy. *Lancet* **1**, 75, 1962.

Ghose, R. (1964) Modern, safe, low cost anaesthesia. *Ethiopian Med. J.* **2**, 221.

Gregory, G. A., Eger, E. I., Smith, N. T., Cullen, B. F. and Cullen, D. J. (1971) Cardiovascular effects of Diethyl Ether in man. *Anesthesiol.* **34**, 19.

Griffith, H. R. and Johnson, G. E. (1942) The use of curare in general anaesthesia. *Anesthesiol.* **3**, 418.

Grogono, A. W. and Porterfield, J. (1970) AMBU valve: Danger of wrong assembly. *Brit. J. Anaesth.* **42**, 978.

Guedel, A. E. (1937) *Inhalation Anaesthesia.* Macmillan, New York.

Haggard, H. W. (1924) The absorption, distribution and elimination of ethyl ether. *J. Biol. Chem.* **59**, 737, 753, 771, 783, 795.

Harrison, G. A. (1964) Ayre's T-piece — a review of its modification. *Brit. J. Anaesth.* **36**, 115.

Hart, S. M. and Bryce-Smith, R. (1963) Cardiac arrhythmias during ether anaesthesia. *Anaesthesia* **18**, 315.

Hjelm, M., Astrup, P., Rörth, M., Verdier, C. H. and Garby, L. (1970) The erythrocyte as a vehicle for oxygen with self-regulating adjustment of unloading. *Scand. J. Clin. Lab. Invest.* **26**, 193.

Holmes, C. McK. (1965) Post-operative vomiting after ether-air anaesthesia. *Anaesthesia* **20**, 199.

Holmes, C. McK. and Bryce-Smith, R. (1964) Halothane as an induction agent. *Anaesthesia* **19**, 399.

Izekono, E., Harmel, M. H. and King, B. D. (1959) Pulmonary ventilation and arterial oxygen saturation during ether-air anesthesia. *Anesthesiol.* **20**, 597.

Jaffe, J. H. (1970) Narcotic Analgesics. In Goodman and Gilman (Eds), *Pharmacological Basis of Therapeutics.* Macmillan, New York.

Jensen, J. K. (1967) Halothankonzentration enreicht durch den "Oxford Miniature Vaporiser". *Der Anaesthesist* **16**, 54.

Johannison, D. (1966) A new non-rebreathing valve. *Acta. Anaesthesiologica. Scand. Suppl.* **26**, 31.

Jones, R. E., Linde, H. W., Deutsch, S., Dripps, R. D. and Price, M. L. (1962) Hemodynamic actions of diethyl ether in normal man. *Anesthesiol.* **23**, 299.

Jorfeldt, L., Löftström, B., Möller, J. and Rósen, A. (1966) Cardiovascular pharmacodynamics of propranolol during ether anaesthesia in man. *Acta. anaesth. Scand. Suppl.* **23**, 263.

Kelly, M. P. (1968) Ventilation equipment (Correspondence). *Brit. Med. J.* 2, 176.

Kelman, G. R. and Kennedy, B. R. (1970) Cardiovascular effects of pancuronium in man. *3rd European Congress of Anaesthesiology Abstracts* 3/02.

Kety, S. S. (1951) The Physiological and Physical factors governing the uptake of anaesthetic gases by the body. *Anesthesiol.* 11, 517.

Khandekar, S. N. and Rama Rao, K. R. (1965) Methoxyflurane in the EMO (Ether) anaesthetic outfit in the armed forces. *Indian J. Anaesth.* 13, 26.

Knight, R. J. (1969) Anaesthesia in a difficult situation in South Vietnam. *Anaesthesia* 24, 317.

Kubota, Y., Schweizer, H. J. and Vandam, L. D. (1962) Hemodynamic effect of diethyl ether in man. *Anesthesiol.* 23, 306.

Latham, J. W. and Parbrook, G. D. (1967) Premixed gas machine. *Anaesthesia* 22, 316.

Leatherdale, R. A. L. (1966) The EMO inhaler: Clinical experience of a thousand anaesthetics. *Anaesthesia* 21, 504.

Lee, J. A. and Atkinson (1968) *Synopsis of anaesthesia.* John Wright, Bristol.

Macintosh, R. R. (1955) A plea for simplicity. *Brit. Med. J.* 2, 1054.

Macintosh, R. R. (1953) Oxford Inflating Bellows. *Brit. Med. J.* 2, 202.

Macintosh, R. R., Mushin, W. W., and Epstein, H. G. (1963) *Physics for the anaesthetist.* Blackwells, Oxford.

Maggio, G. (1962) Betrachtungen über das Wiederbelebungs and Narkosegerät für den Aussendienst. *Der Anaesthesist,* 11, 213.

Maggio, G. and Vogelsanger, G. (1962) L.M.V.B. – Halothane Induction Unit: un nuovo vaporizzatore destinato alla induzione halotanica anche de parte di personale poco qualificato. *Minerva Anest.* 28, 5.

Maklary, E. (1964) Experiences with accurately measurable ether-air anaesthesia. *Proc. 1st. Europ. Cong. Anaesthesiol.* 2, 154.

Mapleson, W. W., Morgan, J. G. and Hillard, E. K. (1963) Assessment of condenser humidifiers with special reference to a multiple gauze model. *Brit. Med. J.* 1, 300.

Markello, R. and King, B. D. (1964) Halothane-ether-air anaesthesia. *J. Amer. Med. Assoc.* 190, 869.

Marshall, B. E. and Grange, R. A. (1966) Changes in respiratory physiology during ether-air anaesthesia. *Brit. J. Anaesth.* 38, 329.

McArdle, L., Black, G. W. and Unni, V. K. N. (1968) Peripheral vascular changes during diethyl ether anaesthesia. *Anaesthesia* 23, 203.

McNally, N. H., Neily, H. H. and Benoit, J. (1962) Anaesthesia for emergency hospitals. *Canad. Anaes. Soc. J.* 9, 524.

Mehta, V., Ratra, C. K., Badola, R. P. and Bhargave, K. P. (1969) Role of different anaesthetic techniques in the incidence of early post-anaesthetic sickness. *Brit. J. Anaesth.* **41**, 689.

Millar, R. A. (1964) EMO Inhaler. *Brit. Med. J.* **1**, 369.

Millar, R. A. and Morris, L. E. (1961) Sympatho-adrenal responses during general anaesthesia in the dog and man. *Canad. Anaesth. Soc. J.* **8**, 356.

Moore, D. C., Bridenbaugh, L. D., Bridenbaugh, P. O. and Tucker, G. T. (1970) Bupivicaine for peripheral nerve block. *Anesthesiol.* **32**, 460.

Morrison, J. D., Clark, R. S. J. and Dundee, J. W. (1970) Studies of drugs given before anaesthesia. XXI: Droperidol. *Brit. J. Anaesth.* **42**, 730.

Moyer, C. A. (1954) *Fluid Balance.* Year Book Medical Publishers, Chicago.

Mushin, W. W., Rendell-Baker, L., Thompson, P. W. and Mapleson, W. W. (1969). *Automatic ventilation of the lungs.* 2nd Edn. Oxford, Blackwell.

Nightingale, F. (1863) *Notes on hospitals* (3rd Edn) London, Longman, Green, Longman, Roberts and Green.

Nunn, J. F. and Freeman, J. (1964) Problems of oxygenation and oxygen transport during haemorrhage. *Anaesthesia* **19**, 206.

Nunn, J. F. and Ezi-Ashi, T. I. (1961) The respiratory effects of resistance to breathing in anaesthetised man. *Anesthesiol.* **35**, 20.

O'Connor, A. P. (1961) Anaesthesia in nuclear warfare. *Irish J. Med. Sci.* **421**, 1.

Oduntan, S. A. (1968) Chloroform Anaesthesia. *Anaesthesia* **23**, 552.

Oduntan, S. A. (1969) Blood gas studies in some abnormal haemoglobins. *W. Afr. Med. J.* **18**, 208.

Parkhouse, J. (1966) Clinical Performance of the O.M.V. inhaler. *Anaesthesia* **21**, 498.

Parkhouse, J. (1960) Genau dosierte Äther-Luft-Narkose für den heutigen Anaesthesisten. *Der Anaesthesist* **9**, 221.

Parkhouse, J., Holmes, C. McK. and Tunstall, M. E. (1963) Anaesthesia with Trichloroethylene and muscle relaxants. *Anaesthesia*, **18**, 482.

Parkhouse, J., Lambrechts, W. and Simpson, B. R. (1961) The incidence of post-operative pain. *Brit. J. Anaesth.* **33**, 345.

Parkhouse, J. and Simpson, B. R. (1959) A restatement of anaesthetic principles. *Brit. J. Anaesth.* **31**, 464.

Pearson, J. W. and Safar, P. (1961) General anaesthesia with minimal equipment. *Anaesth. and Analg.* **40**, 664.

Poppelbaum, H. F. (1960) Rediscovery of air for anaesthesia in thoracic surgery. *Proc. Roy. Soc. Med.* **53**, 289.

Poppelbaum, H. F. and Lutkeholter, G. (1957) Wechseldruckbeatmung ohne CO_2 — Absorptioneinrichtungen in der thoraxchirurgie. *Der Anaesthesist* **6**, 363.

Prior, F. N. (1964) General anaesthesia and analgesia. *J. Chris. Med. Ass. India.* March issue, 1.

Prior, F. N. (1972) Trichloroethylene in air with muscle relaxants. *Anaesthesia* **27**, 66.

Prys-Roberts, C., Kelman, G. R., Greenbaum, R. and Robinson, R. H. (1967) Circulatory influences of artificial respiration during nitrous oxide anaesthesia in man. *Brit. J. Anaesth.* **39**, 533.

Rees, J. G. (1960) Paediatric anaesthesia. *Brit. J. Anaesth.* **32**, 132.

Rigg, D. R. (1961) The present pattern of anaesthetic services in Nigeria. *W. Afr. Med. J.* **10**, 351.

Roth, F. and Wüthrich, H. (1969) The clinical importance of hyperkalaemia following suxamethonium administration. *Brit. J. Anaesth.* **41**, 311.

Scott, D. B. (1968) Inferior vena caval occlusion in late pregnancy and its importance in anaesthesia. *Brit. J. Anaesth.* **40**, 120.

Scott, D. B., Lees, M. M. and Taylor, S. H. (1966) Some respiratory effects of the Trendelenberg position during anaesthesia. *Brit. J. Anaesth.* **38**, 174.

Scott, D. B. and Slawson, K. B. (1968) Respiratory effects of prolonged Trendelenberg position. *Brit. J. Anaesth.* **40**, 103.

Scott, D. L., Pilberg, O. and Vellacott, W. N. (1971) Halothane — Trichloroethylene combination: a re-appraisal. *Brit. J. Anaesth.* **43**, 107.

Sellick, B. A. (1961) Cricoid pressure to control regurgitation of stomach contents during induction of anaesthesia. *Lancet* **2**, 404.

Shires, G. T. and Jackson, D. E. (1962) Postoperative salt tolerance. *Archiv. Surg.* **84**, 703.

Snow, J. (1858) *On chloroform and other anaesthetics.* London, John Churchill.

Snow, J. (1848) On the inhalation of chloroform and ether, with description of apparatus. *Lancet* **1**, 177.

Snow, J. (1847) *On the inhalation of the vapour of ether.* John Churchill, London.

Stephens, K. F. (1963) Some Aspects of anaesthesia in war. *Med. Bull U.S. Army Europe* **20**, 170.

Smith, R. M. (1968) *Anaesthesia for infants and children.* 3rd edition, St. Louis, C. V. Mosby.

Smol'nikov, V. P. (1957) Macintosh's anaesthetic apparatus EMO. *Eksp. Klin.* **2**, 50.

Stetson, J. B. (1968) A simple improvement in the EMO vaporiser. *Brit. J. Anaesth.* **40**, 65.

Stetson, J. B. (1966) The use of the EMO ether vaporiser for paediatric anaesthesia. *Proc. 2nd Europ. Congr. Anaesthesiol.* 503 (*Acta. Anaesth. Scand, Suppl.* 23).

Sugden, J. K. (1970) The use of air in anaesthesia. *Proc. III Asian Australian Congr. Anaesthesiol.* 510.

Sugg, B. R. (1970) EMO vaporiser: Expiratory valves. *Brit. J. Anaesth.* 42, 1024.

Tate, N. (1955) Transillumination of the larynx. *Lancet* 2, 980.

Taylor, W. H. (1970) *Fluid therapy and disorders of electrolyte balance.* Blackwell, Oxford.

Telford, J. and Keats, A. S. (1965) Studies of analgesic drugs, IX. Antagonism of narcotic-induced respiratory depression. *Clin. Pharmacol. Ther.* 6, 12.

Temmerman, P. de. (1960) Methodes d'anesthesie practiques faciles a enseigner rapidement au medecin omnipracticien compte tenu des situations tactiques. *Acta Belg. Arte. Med. Pharm. Milit.* 113, 131.

Tiers, F. M. and Artusio, J. F. (1960) A quantitative study of d-tubocurarine in man during diethyl ether-analgesia. *Anaesthesiol.* 21, 256.

Tunstall, M. E. (1963) Trichloroethylene-Ether-Air. *Anaesthesia* 18, 477.

Vandam, L. D., Schweizer, H. J. and Kubota, Y. (1962) Circulatory response to intra-abdominal manipulation during ether anaesthesia in man. *Circul. Res.* 11, 287.

Volker, R. (1965) A well-controlled inhalation anaesthesia with the EMO inhaler in cats and other animals with a small respiration volume. *Dtsch. tierärztl. Wschr.* 72, 241.

Wade, O. L. and Bishop, J. M. (1962) *Cardiac output and regional blood flow.* Oxford.

Wakai, I. (1963) Human oxygenation by air during anaesthesia: the relation of ventilatory volume and arterial oxygen saturation. *Brit. J. Anaesth.* 35, 414.

Waters, D. J. (1966) Intra-arterial thiopentone (A physico-chemical phenomenon). *Anaesthesia* 21, 346.

Webb, E. (1968) Anaesthesia in primitive conditions. *Canad. Anaes. Soc. J.* 15, 37.

Weis, K. H. and Ahnefeld, F. (1962). Problems of inhalation anaesthesia with simple equipment. *Proc. 1st European Congr. Anaesth.* 82.

Weitzner, S. W., King, B. D. and Izekono, E. (1959) The rate of arterial oxygen desaturation during apnoea in humans. *Anesthesiol.* 20, 624.

Winnie, A. P. and Collins, V. J. (1964) The subclavian perivascular technique of brachial plexus anaesthesia. *Anesthesiol.* 25, 352.

Index